'[This] book provides a comprehensive guide to informed decision-making around well-being, offering valuable insights, shared stories, and resources. This timely contribution seeks to enhance understanding of how health care professionals can better care for themselves while continuing to serve others compassionately.'

Catherine Gamble FRCN, *Nursing Lead Mental Health Programmes, Royal College of Nursing*

I0128443

Workplace Well-Being for Nurses, Health and Care Professionals

This essential guide equips nurses and allied health care professionals with the tools and knowledge for self-care, mindfulness and overall well-being to enable providing compassionate care for others.

Written by a diverse group of contributors who work within the nursing and allied health care fields, this book shares their real-life experiences, expert knowledge, insights and relational-centred practices. Across 11 chapters, the book covers the distinctive pillars of well-being: Physical (regular exercise, sleeping and eating well), Emotional (clinical observation, counselling, peer support, relationships) and Psychological (financial well-being and mental health).

These three pillars of self-care allow readers to address the importance of establishing relational aspects of caring, as a process that requires as much attention as professional practice expertise. For students and practitioners alike, this book delves into important self-care research and applications for healthy personal and sustainable professional lives.

Sally Hardy is closely linked with health and social care, through working with individuals, teams and organisations, promoting practitioner-led inquiry and transformational change through evidence-based health care. Sally's work currently focuses on leading the Norfolk Initiative for Coastal and Rural Health Equalities (NICHE), Anchor Institute within the East of England. Sally's research embraces understanding what factors contribute to sustainable workplace cultures and effective partnerships across health and social care systems. Prior to this, she was Dean of the School of Health Sciences throughout the COVID-19 period. She has also been a non-executive director and continues to promote population and planetary health and well-being through her work internationally.

Workplace Well-Being for Nurses, Health and Care Professionals

EDITED BY
SALLY HARDY

Routledge
Taylor & Francis Group

LONDON AND NEW YORK

Designed cover image: Getty Images | Oxi An

First published 2026
by Routledge
4 Park Square, Milton Park, Abingdon, Oxon OX14 4RN

and by Routledge
605 Third Avenue, New York, NY 10158

Routledge is an imprint of the Taylor & Francis Group, an informa business

British Library Cataloguing-in-Publication Data
A catalogue record for this book is available from the British Library

ISBN: 978-1-041-10147-5 (hbk)
ISBN: 978-1-916-92575-5 (pbk)
ISBN: 978-1-041-05795-6 (ebk)

DOI: 10.4324/9781041057956

Typeset in Vectora LH
by Apex CoVantage, LLC

Contents

List of figures   ix
List of tables   xi
List of contributors   xiii
Foreword   xix

Introduction: Who, how and what can be done to support well-being at work?   1

1 **Health, wealth, and happiness. Is it possible to have it all?**   7
   CARRIE JACKSON

2 **Survival of the workforce**   28
   OSCAR NOEL OCHO

3 **Deep level well-being: Compassion and self-compassion**   48
   ANN JACKSON

4 **Lessons for leading well and living well: A personal reflection**   67
   ALICE WEBSTER

5 **Well-being at work with some homework**   81
   STEVE GREEN AND KATE ROBERTS

6 **Social encounters at work: Sharing is indeed caring**   97
   GEORGIA PANAGIOTAKI, SUSANNE LINDQVIST AND JOEL OWEN

7 **Gambling with health and well-being**   112
   SALLY HARDY

8   In search of meaning through making   129
    JONATHAN WEBSTER AND HOLLY SANDIFORD

9   Staying in the game: Effective strategies for achieving long-
    term career goals   142
    REBEKAH HILL, JULIA HUBBARD AND LORNA SANKEY

10 Eat, drink and be merry; tomorrow we diet   158
    SALLY HARDY

11 Workplace well-being: We are not finished yet   172
    SALLY HARDY

Index   182

Figures

2.1   Developing a Self-Care Plan   40
3.1   The ABC of core work needs   54
5.1   Stepped Psychological Response model   87
6.1   Reflective cycle adapted from Gibbs (1998)   103
7.1   Person-centred gambling severity gauge   120
8.1   'Rock Pool Sculpture' 2020   131
8.2   *Space and Soil* (2023)   135
11.1 Wheel of Life Completed   174

Tables

0.1 Workplace Well-being for Nurses, Health and Care Professionals. Chapter content and author acknowledgements   3

2.1 Factors affecting leadership potentials   33

2.2 Self-assessment tool   41

5.1 Common examples of signs that your well-being is at risk   90

5.2 Common examples of ways to preserve our well-being   91

6.1 Barriers and facilitators identified from introducing interprofessional Schwartz Rounds in the higher education setting   107

7.1 Gambling treatment options: a comparison of the evidence   118

10.1 Brown's STRENGTH mnemonic for healthy living   168

Contributors

Steve Green is working as Consultant Clinical NeuroPsychologist at Lincolnshire Partnership NHS Trust, having previously led the innovative staff well-being service at the Queen Elizabeth Hospital, Kings Lynn.

Sally Hardy is Director of NICHE Anchor Institute for Norfolk and Waveney ICS, Faculty of Medicine and Health Sciences, University of East Anglia, engaging internationally to promote highly effective integrated health care focused on those most at risk of inequalities. Throughout her academic career, Professor Sally Hardy has remained closely linked with the NHS, promoting practitioner-led inquiry and transformational change through evidence-based health care. Sally re-joined the University of East Anglia in September 2019 as Professor of Mental Health and Practice Innovation and was Dean of the School of Health Sciences throughout the COVID-19 pandemic, working in collaboration with the East of England Deans of Health. She is now focusing on leading the Norfolk Initiative for Coastal and Rural Health Equalities (NICHE), Anchor Institute for the Norfolk and Waveney Integrated Care System (ICS) and is Chair of the Eastern Partnership for Innovation in Integrated Care (EPIIC) across six Higher Education Institutions and associated ICSs across the East of England. Sally's research focuses on understanding what factors contribute to sustainable workplace cultures and effective health and social care systems. In collaboration with Norwich University of Arts, the Restoration Trust and other local partners is a founding member of the Norfolk Arts and Health Collaborative. She is also a founding member of the annual Skellern Lecture series, and manages the annual Worshipful Company of Barbers, Nursing Clinical Scholarships. She has recently achieved Freedom of the City of London for her contribution as a nurse, and acknowledged as the Skellern Lifetime Achievement awardee 2025.

Rebekah Hill is Associate Professor of Nursing in the School of Health Sciences at the University of East Anglia, where she works as the Assessment Lead. Rebekah worked as a nurse within Gastroenterology and Hepatology, Critical Care and Acute Medicine for many years, completing her PhD on the experience of living with hepatitis C.

Julia Hubbard is Emeritus Professor of Clinical Health Education at the University of East Anglia and a highly experienced academic having worked in university-level health care education since 1993. Her expertise includes undergraduate and postgraduate curriculum development and course delivery across a range of health care professions both nationally and internationally. Her academic roles have included working as Head of Department for Nursing, Midwifery and Nurse Apprenticeships, which involved managing a large academic team across a wide range of Nursing and Midwifery Council (NMC) approved programmes. She was also the Director of International Partnerships for the School of Health Sciences, UEA, supporting student travel abroad and fostering working and research partnerships with health science schools across the globe.

Ann Jackson has been working as a registered mental health nurse for over four decades, with interests and roles primarily focused on practice development in mental health, women's mental health, violence against women and girls and suicide prevention. Ann has led a national programme of practice development in mental health, working with NHS and private provider teams, working as an external facilitator to integrate best contemporary mental health nursing evidence and policy. She established the Royal College of Nursing's Women's Mental Health Group and worked at the Department of Health supporting the development of policy for women in the criminal justice system. She was Director of Nursing at St. Andrew's Healthcare, the largest UK charitable provider of specialist mental health services, and in 2015, she accepted a year's interim post of Deputy Director of Nursing for NHS England (Central Midlands). From 2016, working as Independent and Associate Consultant, Ann has designed and delivered bespoke workshops, learning sets and leadership programmes to develop political awareness, wholehearted and compassionate leadership. Her leadership facilitation approach supports senior nurses and clinical health care professionals explore and develop their skills to create a culture of psychological safety where compassionate and collective leadership can be bravely curated. As lead for suicide prevention within an NHS Trust, Ann became more committed to guided support and self-compassion to genuinely protect the well-being of staff working in challenging and emotionally demanding contexts. Over the years, she has worked with ward leaders, clinical team leaders, matrons and band 8 clinical or system leaders. Over the last eight years, Ann has also worked effectively co-facilitating for the Foundation of Nursing Studies: (FoNS) Creating Caring Cultures Across Mental Health and Learning Disability Services in Northern Ireland; Hilary McCallion Consultancy

Ltd: Leadership in Care Programmes and NICHE at the University of East Anglia: 'Leading and Facilitating the Development of Person-Centred Care and Cultures'. All programmes are provided in partnership with NHS providers of mental health. This last programme involved a five-day residential programme, supported for a following year with group and 1:1 education, support and coaching with Ann. Finally, as a facilitator and coach, Ann draws on her breadth of leadership experiences and wisdom to develop trusting relationships, strengthening lines of awareness and understanding, providing contemporary knowledge to actively support leaders fully embody their role as leaders with optimum influence and impact. She offers team and 1:1 coaching for compassionate and impactful leadership.

Carrie Jackson is Visiting Senior Fellow at the University of East Anglia. She has an extensive portfolio of multiprofessional curriculum design, and leadership roles in higher education and the NHS spanning 35+ years. She has previously been Research Director for several research centres at UEA and was the founding co-director of the England Centre for Practice Development and member of the International Practice Development Collaborative (IPDC). A nurse by background, she is passionate about making a difference in practice working with all the professions to improve the quality of person-centred safe and effective care and services. Her recent interests are in community well-being and flourishing through social innovation and entrepreneurship, working with neighbourhoods to help address some of the major issues affecting health and well-being posed by recent world events. She works with a range of creative practitioners from the arts and humanities, using creative media to help support inclusion and participation of vulnerable groups in our communities. She holds a number of visiting positions internationally.

Susanne Lindqvist is Director of the Centre for Interprofessional Practice (CIPP) and Professor of Interprofessional Practice. She is also Director of Educational strategy, Learning and Teaching Quality at Norwich Medical School (NMS). The purpose of CIPP initiative was to give students an opportunity to learn with, from and about each other, allowing them to develop knowledge, skills, attitudes, values and behaviour that underpin effective interprofessional practice and high-quality care across twelve different professions. Working together with others both locally, nationally and internationally has been a key ingredient in CIPP's and Susanne's approach to finding the best way forward in the joint attempt at providing meaningful opportunities for learning and working together that lead to real improvements in patient/client care. In October 2019, Susanne became an EMCC accredited coach for senior leaders so that she can actively help promote the overall aim of CIPP by supporting people to develop and optimise their leadership skills.

Oscar Noel Ocho started his career as Nursing Assistant Trainee at San Fernando
General Hospital in 1981. As a qualified RN, he currently serves as Director, University
of the West Indies School of Nursing (UWISoN), St Augustine, as well as Director, PAHO/
WHO Collaborating Centre (Nursing Leadership and Policy). He was a public servant
for 34 years prior to joining the Faculty at UWI. Dr Ocho is Population Leadership
Fellow, University of Washington, and a Caribbean Health Leadership Institute Scholar.
A member of the Member Commission on Graduates of Foreign Nursing Schools
(CGFNS) International Global Health Workforce Development Institute Advisory
Committee, he has 24 peer-reviewed publications, four book chapters and 199 citations.
His research interests include health systems, leadership and gender and health.

Joel Owen is Associate Professor and Psychological Well-being Practitioner (PWP)
Programme Director, in the Department of Clinical Psychology and Psychological
Therapies (CPPT), Norwich Medical School, University of East Anglia. The main
focus of Joel's research is on the topic of well-being, having worked on multiple
projects related to this for several years, and it is also the topic of his PhD. His clinical
background is as a PWP, having trained at UEA before working over a period of
several years in two separate IAPT services in the East of England. His academic
background before training in IAPT was in philosophy, bringing together his passions
for philosophy and psychology in practice ways, human flourishing and resilience, as
well as the philosophical origins of Cognitive Behavioural Therapies (CBT).

Georgia Panagiotaki is Associate Professor with a background in Developmental
Psychology, who teaches on Developmental and Health Psychology, Consultation
Skills and Evidence-Based Medicine in the undergraduate medical course at UEA
(MBBS). As lead for the psychology theme, she is responsible for the design and
delivery of the psychology and well-being curriculum in the MBBS. Georgina is
the well-being lead for the MBBS course, working closely with the school's senior
advising team, the faculty's embedded team and university student services to
support students' well-being and increase awareness around student mental
health and well-being, leading UEA's Interprofessional Student Schwartz Rounds,
an initiative recently introduced to all health professional undergraduate and
postgraduate courses at UEA. Her developmental psychology research has evolved
from the study of children's conceptual development in the domain of astronomy
(the topic of my DPhil) to the study of children's understanding of biology, the
human body and the concepts of life, health, illness and death, understanding
how these concepts develop and how culture and culturally specific experiences
influence children's reasoning in this domain.

Kate Roberts is Principal Clinical Psychologist, Department of Clinical Health
Psychology at the Queen Elizabeth Hospital King's Lynn NHS Foundation Trust. She

works to promote psychological well-being through her research and active clinical work. As a psychologist, a big part of Kate's role is supporting people to live a fulfilling life alongside pain. Everyone has different life experiences, and no two people's pain is quite alike, so hearing people's stories and working alongside them to consider how to improve their quality of life has become an important aspect of her clinical specialism.

Holly Sandiford is an artist, educator and researcher with over 25 years of experience in arts and well-being. Her work explores the relationships between people, place and the natural world, using photography, sound and mixed media. As co-director of ArtatWork CIC, she develops projects that connect creativity with mental health and community well-being. She is also a researcher at Norwich University of the Arts and works with UEA NICHE and Norfolk Museums Service to explore the impact of arts and heritage on well-being. Holly has led workshops, exhibitions and commissions for museums, universities and cultural organisations, including the Fitzwilliam Museum, hospital rooms and Leicester Space Park.

Lorna Sankey is a registered occupational therapist, and works as a senior research associate. Her time at UEA covered working to explore the impact of workplace well-being on the nursing workforce.

Alice Webster has been Chief Executive of the Queen Elizabeth Hospital NHS Foundation Trust, King's Lynn, England. As Registered General Nurse and Midwife and subsequently Health Visitor in the early 1990s, Alice has worked in both secondary and primary care in the UK and Australia. With over 30 years' experience in nursing and leadership, latterly with 15 years in executive leadership and management, Alice is attuned to the challenges that individuals may have working in large complex systems, ensuring the patient voice remains core to the delivery of services. Having held three chief nurse positions within three different NHS Regions, Alice has experience working across acute, community, mental health and ambulance services. She uses her learning to inform, nurture, develop and grow underpinned by the importance of authenticity in which people and communities are central. Alice has developed a skills set that is able to guide an organisation or professional group towards its goals by setting vision, developing strategy, managing current and aspiring new talent whilst shaping context and culture that is both collaborative, creative and transformational.

Jonathan Webster is Professor of Practice Development and Co-Director, Norfolk Initiative for Coastal and Rural Health Equalities (NICHE) – Anchor Institute, University of East Anglia. Jonathan's career stretches over 30+ years working for the NHS and across Higher Education. As a registered general nurse, he has worked in both secondary and community settings in the UK and

Australia. His clinical practice expertise is older people's nursing, having held two Consultant Nurse posts for Older People. During this time, he led programmes of education, practitioner-centred research, evaluation and practice development, having held honorary gerontological and practice development fellowships with the Royal College of Nursing Institute. In 2011 Jonathan became North West London PCTs Cluster Director of Nursing and Quality, before becoming the Director of Quality and Nursing for five of the CCGs. Between July 2017 and August 2019, he was seconded to NHS England/Improvement initially in the London Region as Director of Nursing and latterly in the South East Region as Interim Regional Chief Nurse. Joining UEA in July 2020, Jonathan joined NICHE when it formed in January 2023. He has been involved in national and international work related to older persons' care; practice and system development; workplace culture; quality improvement and leadership. Jonathan's professional interests lie in developing person-centred cultures of practice that enable those involved in health and care to work in partnership with people and communities through practice development, service transformation and action research.

Foreword

'Beneath our clothes, our reputations, our pretensions, beneath our religion or lack of it, we are all vulnerable both to the storm without and to the storm within'.

Frederick Buechner's poignant excerpt from *Telling the Truth* reminds us that beneath our roles, reputations, and pretensions, we are all susceptible to challenges both external and internal. This universal vulnerability extends to health care professionals, who share the common humanity of their patients. Compassion and connection remain at the heart of health care values, regardless of who is affected by ill health, when or where it occurs.

Despite the centrality of compassion, health care professionals face mounting pressures. Operating within disadvantaged communities with limited resources while managing complex cases demands emotional resilience and adaptability. This truth, though often unspoken, forms the bedrock of empathy in the caring professions. When we acknowledge the shared fragility that underpins every human interaction, we invite greater honesty and openness – qualities vital to both seeking help and offering support.

Paradoxically, the expectation often placed on health care professionals to maintain these values can lead them to neglect their own well-being. The reluctance to share personal vulnerabilities and carry on regardless further compounds the strain.

Nursing is widely acknowledged as a demanding career, and in recent years there has been a noticeable rise in nurses needing time off due to depression, anxiety, stress, or other mental health concerns. Although employers have a legal responsibility to protect staff from workplace stress, increasing levels of sick leave, early retirement, and staff resignations continue to be reported.

In 2019, whilst I was the RCN Professional Lead for Mental Health, the RCN Foundation commissioned the Society for Occupational Medicine (SOM) to conduct a study into the Mental Health and Well-being of Nurses and Midwives in the UK: Prevalence, Risk Factors, Implications and Interventions. Their report highlighted that challenging, critical working environments play a significant role in the mental health struggles and burnout experienced by nurses and midwives. Conducted before the COVID-19 pandemic, the study found that excessive workloads, poor leadership, lack of resources, and workplace bullying not only threatened nurses' well-being but also hindered organisations to retain their staff and their ability to deliver safe, high-quality patient care.

Unlike most physical health issues, the signs of mental health decline can be subtle and easy to miss; all too often, rather than being understood, the symptoms can be criticised and personalised. Colleagues may not notice or act on early warning signs. They may be ill advised, but they aren't alone. As a mental health nurse with 30+ years of clinical experience, I have worked with many patients' families from all communities, who retrospectively recall changes in attitudes, beliefs, and behaviours that they wished they had aired concerns about, sought help for or talked through when initially noticed. There is a need to nurture a climate where well-being is prioritised, and health care professionals feel less isolated by the burdens they bear.

Professor Sally Hardy and her colleagues have recognised these challenges and created a much-needed resource. Their book provides a comprehensive guide to informed decision-making around well-being, offering valuable insights, shared stories, and resources. This timely contribution seeks to enhance understanding of how health care professionals can better care for themselves while continuing to serve others compassionately.

Promoting self-care and understanding among health care workers is essential in navigating the demands of modern health care systems. By addressing vulnerabilities and prioritizing well-being, professionals can ensure that they sustain the values of compassion and care in their work, even amidst the complexities of today's health care environment.

Catherine Gamble
Royal College Nursing Fellow

Introduction
Who, how and what can be done to support well-being at work?

WELL-BEING IN THE WORKPLACE

When considering how to construct a book focused on workplace well-being it was important to recognise that we each approach life and its associated difficulties differently. Our uniqueness is influenced by our upbringing, genetic makeup and life experiences. All these elements work to shape us, make us or indeed sometimes conspire to break us, or rather to remold us.

Well-being at work is potentially something you have not had to think about. It is indeed a difficult subject. It may have been something thrust upon you, whether due to a dramatic change in personal circumstances, relating to either poor health, poor workplace practices, stress of workplace redundancies, the impact of organisational re-structures or any other stressful life event that we all must face from time to time. Yet the purpose of this book is to help you navigate working life and to maximise your ability to transcend many of life's complex difficulties. It is not a book of policies and procedures. It is more a discipline, exploring workplace well-being as a process of self-discovery. It is also about shared knowledge, and self-awakening to how we work well, starting with self, as a guide to living and working well in the modern complex and stressful world of health and social care, as professional caregivers. The book aims to capture a difficult life path we all take. Yet facing the fact that life is indeed difficult is in itself a first step to addressing our workplace well-being, as outlined by Peck (1978) who states:

> Life is difficult. This is a great truth, one of the greatest truths. . . . Once we truly understand and accept it – then life is no longer difficult. Because once it is accepted, the fact that life is difficult no longer matters.
>
> (Peck, 1978; p 15)

DOI: 10.4324/9781041057956-1

This book has been written by colleagues, whose contributions ensure each chapter is based upon their professional research interests, personal experiences and from a collective desire to share their learnings as health and care professionals from across diverse and varied careers.

When bringing these chapters together, the focus is on how these unique experiences, expressed in the different chapters, can help you consider what, how and who needs to be involved in securing and maximising your well-being, both at work and at home.

Each chapter can be explored in isolation. Dipping into the features will bring the ideas alive, through case study examples and learning resources, for you to investigate and develop further, or to share these insights with your colleagues, teams or family members. The chapters are also intertwined so you can read each of them methodically, as concepts of our mental and physical health, wealth and happiness are looked at from different perspectives. Some explore personal workplace experience and well-being potentials, whilst others focus on professional opportunities to advance your health and well-being longevity.

Chapter content

In capturing what and where opportunities are available to maximise your own, your colleagues', and indeed patients' health and well-being, each chapter of this book will be one that will come as a welcome relief in times of need, but also useful as a highly effective prevention strategy in promoting healthy, happy lives as health and care professionals, both in the workplace and at home in your personal leisure time.

Chapter 1 explores some fundamental concepts of health, wealth, and happiness in terms of whether we can really have it all. What is happiness anyway, and does seeking promotion and more money really bring satisfaction? This chapter outlines work Carrie has achieved with others in facilitating workplace cultures of effectiveness, using the workplace as a place for learning, where everyone's contribution is taken into consideration to make improvements together.

Chapter 2 takes these ideas further, in terms of what and how to promote the necessary leadership skills and requirements of self-efficacy, from which to translate skills of leadership across multiple organisations. Chapter 2 also pays attention to understanding the demands of leadership from different staff groups, and from the people encountered inside and external to the workplace. Oscar's chapter is built upon work and experience gained from a lengthy career spanning

Table 0.1 Workplace Well-being for Nurses, Health and Care Professionals. Chapter content and author acknowledgements

Chapter	Title	Author(s)
Intro	Who, how and what can be done to support well-being at work?	Sally Hardy
1	Health, wealth, and happiness. Is it possible to have it all?	Carrie Jackson
2	Survival of the workforce	Oscar Noel Ocho
3	Deep level well-being: Compassion and self-compassion	Ann Jackson
4	Lessons for leading well and living well: A personal reflection	Alice Webster
5	Well-being at work with some homework	Steve Green and Kate Roberts
6	Social encounters at work: Sharing is indeed caring	Georgia Panagiotaki, Susanne Lindqvist and Joel Owen
7	Gambling with health and well-being	Sally Hardy
8	In search of meaning through making	Jonathan Webster and Holly Sandiford
9	Staying in the game: Effective strategies for achieving longterm career goals	Rebekah Hill, Julia Hubbard and Lorna Sankey
10	Eat, drink and be merry; tomorrow we diet	Sally Hardy
11	Workplace well-being: We are not finished yet	Sally Hardy

Source: **Sally Hardy**

the Caribbean, USA and England workplace contexts and cultures. Self-efficacy is explored as a way of measuring and reflecting on how to remain authentic, which includes remaining open to new ways of considering what influences our effectiveness in the workplace.

Chapter 3 takes the concept of authentic leadership further into the realms of compassionate interactions with self and others. Ann shares her commitment to considering leadership from a coaching and enablement perspective. Her work on suicide prevention offers access to some world-class tool kits and resources.

In Chapter 4, Alice provides another perspective on leading well. How the experiences of a leader who remains authentic can sometimes prove an isolating experience if not balanced well with self-care and a workplace context that embraces humane values and beliefs.

Chapter 5 explores how providing a workplace staff support service brings into focus what place the organisation has for staff, particularly since the consequences of the COVID-19 pandemic and impact on workforce resilience and well-being has been, and continues to be felt as, hard hitting. Steve and Kate share their learnings from an approach developed in a rural district hospital, where spreading the notion of psychological first aiders also helped manage the rising demands of workplace well-being.

Chapter 6 looks specifically at another workplace intervention, in using Schwartz Rounds, for enhancing ability to safely explore emotional responses to difficult and challenging work situations with our colleagues. Suzanne and colleagues share the work these Rounds offer to prepare students for the emotional realm of working in health and social care.

The book then moves to explore more personal well-being approaches and the impact this might have on workplace effectiveness and our personal mental and physical well-being, to consider how sustainability can be achieved from a starting point of self-care and self-compassion.

Chapter 7 explores one of those topics not often discussed openly at work. I explore gambling, in terms of what it means to our health and well-being, and how it manifests. As health and care professionals, do we take our health and well-being for granted, gambling with ours and others' health, as if we are immune to damage incurred?

Chapter 8 offers an example of balancing workplace activities with undertaking mindful practices that bring us health and well-being. Jonathan and Holly share their experience of making meaning through creative expression. Many of you, I hope, will find meaning, and might even spark some creative activities and hobbies of your own, perhaps that have been laid aside due to pressures of work and study, life- and work-related time constraints.

Chapter 9 is about 'staying in the game', in terms of how we ensure our careers are long and sustainable. Rebekah and colleagues share work they have been doing to improve approaches to retaining staff, as highly effective retention strategies, which are often overlooked in workforce strategy planning.

In Chapter 10, I take us back to look again at how we look after ourselves, in terms of decisions, habits and behaviours associated with what we eat, our sleep patterns and level of physical as well as mental health. Some motivation tools and examples for improving and moving from good intentions to forming healthy lifetime habits are shared as part of the learning resources this book has captured throughout.

The concluding Chapter 11 is where I attempt to bring the book to a conclusion and summarise the collective learning achieved across all the chapters. The intention is to encourage you to use what you have read to promote an active interest in self-care and kindness. A summative checklist is offered for you to use, and add to, as your self-discovery of workplace well-being continues.

HOW TO USE THIS BOOK?

An introduction section outlines the chapter focus and gives you an indication of how the author(s) have structured the chapter content.

Each brings a case study, to really bring to life the issues being discussed within them. All have lengthy references, showing how our work is steeped in current practices and contemporary evidence that you can go and investigate further.

Each has a series of additional materials, posing questions for self-reflection and discovery.

A further reading and resources available section will help to take your learning back to your teams and colleagues, as exercises or ideas for team building, and introducing more workplace well-being strategies.

Finally, each chapter has captured the references used to back up what is being said in the chapter. Again, this can be used for you to further explore the literature on a subject.

I hope this becomes a useful resource to you and something you can use repeatedly, to challenge yourself to be as healthy, happy and a highly effective, authentic human being.

Sally

REFERENCE

Peck, M. S. (1978). *The road less traveled: A new psychology of love, traditional values and spiritual growth*. Simon & Schuster.

Chapter 1

Health, wealth, and happiness. Is it possible to have it all?

Carrie Jackson

INTRODUCTION

In this first chapter the interrelationship between key concepts of health, wealth and happiness, their theoretical foundations, and their impact on well-being and quality of life are explored. Achieving health, wealth, and happiness is a complex and deeply personal pursuit. All three are interconnected and play a crucial role in our overall well-being. While it is possible to balance these elements, it often requires careful planning, consistent effort, and mindfulness. But is it really possible to have it all?

Different life experiences will be presented. Starting from a global financial and public policy macro perspective, then a meso-perspective in the workplace, and then through our personal lives and the values we hold dear – at a micro perspective. Strategies to improve our overall health, well-being, and happiness through self-care are shared. The latter point is particularly important because as a health professional, caring for self will ensure that you are effective in caring for others, both in your personal and professional life.

DEFINING HEALTH, WEALTH, AND HAPPINESS

Physical and mental well-being are important health foundations for achieving both wealth and happiness.

The World Health Organization defines *health* as "a state of complete physical, mental and social well-being and not merely the absence of disease or infirmity" (WHO, 1948). A good healthy state, in mind and body, increases

DOI: 10.4324/9781041057956-2

productivity, focus, and energy, enabling you to achieve life goals and enjoy life to the full.

Dictionary definitions of *wealth* generally describe an abundance of money, property, or other valuable assets considered important to the individual. This might be knowledge; e.g., a person has a *wealth of knowledge*, or skills, or a rich and varied lived experience. A person's financial stability can provide security and opportunities for pursuing passions, which in turn can enhance happiness. However, an obsession with accumulating wealth can lead to stress, burnout, and social imbalance, diminishing health and joy.

Financial stability is an important aspect of life, as it gives you the freedom to live the life you want without having to worry about money. Learning to create a budget and saving regularly is about investing in your future. It is also important to live within your means and avoid debt whenever possible. Financial advice is often freely available, from a bank, building society, or charities, such as spending a small amount on getting a financial advisor, which is another investment in oneself. However, consider this early so that any capital is used wisely, to cover for any of life's unexpected challenges through a financial plan for retirement, or for your family's future (school trips and university fees, etc.)

A long-running American study at Harvard University (since 1938) followed 700 men and their spouses across three generations. They found that participants with more prestigious jobs, and therefore more money, were no happier in their lives. The point is to not treat money as the ultimate goal, but as a means to an end, to shape a meaningful existence. If not, life has the potential to pass us all by, and happiness is something we can put off into the future that may never be attained.

> *Money can't buy us happiness, but it's a tool that can give us security and safety and a sense of control over lives. At the end of the day, life is really about our connections with others. It's our relationships that keep us happy.*
> (Waldinger and Shculzm, 2023, p 22)

The Harvard Study of Adult Development reveals that the strength of our connections with others can predict the health of both our bodies and our brains as we go through life (Waldinger and Shculzm, 2023).

HAPPINESS

Happiness is a multi-dimensional concept made up of several constructs which include affective well-being (feelings of joy and pleasure), eudaimonic well-being (sense of meaning and purpose in life), and evaluative well-being (life satisfaction)

(Steptoe et al 2015). According to Steptoe (2019) the relationship between happiness and health is developing rapidly, exploring the possibility that impaired happiness is not only a consequence of ill-health but also a potential contributor to disease risk.

Happiness may be experienced as both a temporary emotional state (feeling happy in the moment) and a more enduring sense of well-being (being satisfied with life). A sense of fulfilment can come from personal relationships, meaningful work, or leisure pursuits. It is defined in various ways, depending on the perspective from which you are examining it. There are other frameworks also identified in the further reading section.

Historically happiness has been studied by a number of philosophers, psychologists, and economists, expanding our knowledge of how happiness can be measured, what factors contribute to it, and how individuals and societies can cultivate well-being. There are more frameworks to look at in the further reading section.

HOW DOES GLOBAL PUBLIC POLICY AND ECONOMICS IMPACT THE MANAGEMENT OF A PERSON'S HEALTH, WEALTH, AND HAPPINESS?

Happiness is considered important as a predictor of world health that the United Nations (UN) General Assembly invited all member countries to measure happiness from 2011 annually and use it to help guide public policy; the Assembly initiated the World Happiness Report, which provides an annual league table of happiness across countries. The UN comments that social environments influencing happiness are diverse and interwoven, differing within and among communities, nations, and cultures. However the World Happiness Report (UN 2019: 31) states that having someone to count on, trust (as measured by the absence of corruption), a sense of freedom to make key life decisions, and generosity together account for as much as the combined effects of income and healthy life expectancy in explaining the life evaluation gap between the ten happiest and the ten least happy countries in the world.

Governments cannot control every aspect of personal happiness, but by creating environments where citizens' basic needs are met, opportunities for personal growth and fulfilment are available, and social trust is high, which can foster a generally happier society. While happiness is subjective, governments can address factors that contribute to overall societal contentment. Many Western governments provide accessible universal healthcare services, ensuring citizens can maintain a good standard of physical and mental health without excessive financial burden. Political influence focuses on financial stability by ensuring employment opportunities, monitoring and setting fair wages, and offering unemployment benefits to help reduce burden of financial stress and insecurity. Social safety nets such as welfare programs, pensions, and healthcare subsidies protect vulnerable populations to reduce poverty.

Public health programs help to promote healthy lifestyles, offer a preventive approach to health and associated mental health, which works towards a happier, healthier society. Mental health public policies that provide support and access counselling and mental health services are key. Governments that prioritise mental health, reduce stigma, and provide adequate services can alleviate the psychological burdens on citizens, contributing to higher happiness levels. Accessible high-quality education and lifelong learning from early childhood to higher education empowers people, enhances job opportunities, and fosters personal development, all contributing to a person's state of happiness.

Another government-driven approach includes developing policies that promote healthy work-life balance, through regulating working hours and conditions. Countries like Norway and Denmark, with shorter average working hours and strong labour protections, often rank highly in happiness due to a focus on achieving a healthy work-life balance. Family leave policies which include paid maternity/paternity leave, vacation time, and sick leave can help to reduce stress and promote happiness by supporting time with family and on personal well-being, such as spending time outside, in the green and blue spaces of your local landscape.

Countries that focus on environmental sustainability often also rank highly in happiness rates. Government Environmental Policies for sustainable development and urban planning can also help to promote clean air, protect green and blue spaces through environmental protections which directly impact well-being and health. Building liveable cities with access to nature, recreation, and cultural spaces promotes happiness by improving quality of life. Supporting cultural initiatives, arts, and community events fosters a sense of identity, belonging, connection and brings joy, as people celebrate together. Policies that encourage the building of community, through for example social support networks and public spaces where people can gather, promotes social interaction and reduces isolation, which increases happiness. Strong social ties, wealth and a variety of support systems are associated with overall states of happiness.

WORKPLACE CULTURE

Given we spend around one-third of our lives at work, or just under 90,000 hours over our lifetime (Office of National Statistics 2021 Census), it is important that work is both productive and fulfilling. How and what we experience in the workplace impacts our personal health and well-being, as well as our financial goals, career, and life aspirations.

CASE STUDY

A team of clinicians working in an acute hospital were experiencing a high turnover of staff, and dealing with some difficult patients with multiple, life-threatening illnesses. The families of these patients were often hanging about the ward, watching what was going on with very high levels of anxiety and concern for their loved ones. Staff were feeling watched, criticised from all sides, and were not working well as a team. One staff member refused to work on the same shifts as some colleagues, others were actively looking for jobs elsewhere and speaking openly, in front of patients, about benefits of seeking a job in their local supermarket, so at least they could get reduced food bills and other perks they did not get here. Any staff vacancies were not easily being filled. And when new, or temporary, staff did arrive, they rarely stayed.

The ward manager invited an external facilitator to help address the workplace culture, that had become bullying, backstabbing, and with high levels of staff sickness. The first meeting explored the background of what had been happening to the team, as a self-assessment of their context and situation. The ward manager and I then moved to planning how to engage staff and patients, in a process of workplace culture mapping.

Following several visits to the staff team meetings, a plan was identified to address several co-designed small projects, and to obtain feedback from patients and families. We also agreed to invite other colleagues outside the ward team, to attend an observation of practice period and provide feedback of what they saw, felt, and heard. Staff were both highly sceptical of what this extra work would produce, but eventually, after a period of capturing their own thoughts, ideas, and experiences, became quite excited at the possibilities, and agreed a way forward, as a shared purpose and vision for the ward team, and identified new ways of working together as a functioning team.

Several months later, even though several staff had resigned and moved on, those remaining began to influence some practical changes. Patients noticed the atmosphere on the ward became mellow. There was less shouting, frenetic running about, and a more focused attention being given to conversations between the team, and with patients, including their families, instead of asking them to leave the room. If time was to be offered, it was planned, so that challenges were addressed as a team, with agreed next steps implemented, evaluated, and improvement noted. Gradually, the ward became known for its innovation and a supportive, engaged clinical team. The vacancies were filled, and a process of ongoing improvements with some ambitious plans for painting, decorating, and undertaking research began to take place, as people's confidence and respect for each other grew.

An effective workplace culture is one that is experienced as providing a safe and effective environment. In health and social care settings, a workplace culture that can enhance the health and Wellbeing of staff and service users alike, is identified as a place where peoples contributions are both recognised and valued.

(Manley et al, 2014)

It is underpinned by values of respect for persons (personhood), individual right to self-determination, mutual respect, and understanding. It is enabled by cultures of empowerment that foster continuous approaches to practice development.

(McCormack and McCance 2017, p 3)

SHARED PURPOSE

A workplace that has a shared purpose unites people in shared decision making and enables and empowers people to collaborate effectively working in the same direction around a set of agreed values and ways of working that get the best out of each other's skills, talents, and interests so that challenges and barriers can be overcome together (Manley et al 2014; Manley et al 2011a, 2011b). Having a sense of shared purpose, being clear about contributions through role clarity, and having the necessary competence to be able to fulfil the job role effectively, within a supportive environment, is important for personal and professional development, leading to improved happiness and well-being.

Purpose taps into people's need for meaningful work; to be part of something bigger than ourselves. It encapsulates people's cognitive, emotional and spiritual commitment to a cause. . . . Purpose becomes shared when we find commonalities between our values, beliefs and aspirations.

(Finney, 2013, p 6)

The consequences of working in a positive workplace culture are continuous evidence that the needs of patients, users and communities are met in a person centred way; staff are empowered, happy and committed; standards, goals and objectives are met; and knowledge/evidence is developed, used and shared in a way that enables everyone to flourish.

(Manley et al 2011a, 2011b)

ADDRESSING WORKPLACE STRESSORS

Workload and job-related stressors for health and social care workers has increased, through, for example, long working hours and unsocial working patterns, consequence of COVID-19, a backlog of treatment waiting lists, coupled with the complex multiple demands of an increasingly ageing population, and medical, health, and social care workforce shortages in Western countries (Shiri et al 2023, Hill et al 2022, Li et al 2021, Ghahramani et al 2023, Sheldon et al 2008). High levels of stress and heavy workload can lead to a higher risk of burnout, stress, insomnia, anxiety, depression (Ghahramani et al 2023), physical and mental ill-health, and an inability to work (Romero-Sanchez et al 2022).

In order to tackle workplace stressors, it is important that employers implement effective interventions in the workplace that can reduce physical and psychosocial risk factors, improve working conditions, and enhance employees health and well-being (Shiri et al 2023). Examples cited in the literature as being effective for improving employee mind and body well-being include group or team-based activities such as the following:

- Mindfulness-based cognitive therapy (Spinelli et al 2019; Lomas et al 2018), an eight-week mindfulness-based stress reduction intervention (van Dijk et al 2017), and unguided digital mindfulness-based self-practices (Taylor et al 2022). Practicing mindfulness and relaxation; e.g., meditation, deep breathing, or yoga, for example, can help manage stress and improve mental clarity (Perez et al 2017).

- Group physical exercises, such as supervised high-intensity workplace strengthening exercises plus group coaching (Jakobsen et al 2015), or a six-week supervised workplace exercise programme involving stretching, strengthening, aerobic and balance exercises (Gerodimos et al 2022), and an intervention to enhance coping with job demand and/or to boost job resources (Müller et al 2016).

It is not possible to provide an exhaustive list of all of the tools policies and practices that might be employed in the workplace, but Table 1.5 in the further reading section gives some examples of where to start. If you do not use any of these already, perhaps start with a self-assessment, to identify your strengths and areas for development, and then check these out with your peers. Inviting feedback is an important part of your reflective career development and self-assessment process, helping to keep focused and self-critique in balance. This will also help to create a personal development plan and SMART (specific, measurable, achievable, realistic, and timed) personal and professional career objectives. Such a holistic reflective approach helps you to stay grounded and focused and avoid feeling overwhelmed. This approach can also be useful evidence from which to base discussions with a workplace mentor or coach and bring to your line manager during your annual appraisal.

Reflecting on your own happiness at work, or at home, is key to understanding yourself, your values, what is important to you, and what you hope to achieve in life, all of which contributes to creating work-life balance and personal well-being. Use the following questions to consider a self-reflection on the following aspects of your work-life balance and future plans.

Reflection

- Career success does not always equate to your happiness. What other activities bring you joy, excitement, and a sense of fulfilment?
- Treasure work relationships, because we spend a lot of time at work, and those relationships are important to our well-being. Who at work are you key supporters, as someone whose opinion you value?
- Prepare a post-retirement life plan early. This helps to build a life framework with purpose and meaning.
- What are the support networks you have outside of work? Do you need to take up new or old hobbies? When do you have time to focus on close, meaningful friendships? Have you, or do you, need to build a series of support networks outside of work?

- Value experiences over things; rather than accumulating possessions (bigger house, faster car), use your money to share experiences with others; e.g., a holiday, treating friends to a nice dinner, charitable giving, volunteering your time and skills to those less fortunate.

SELF-CARE

Choosing behaviours which help you balance the effects of physical and emotional stress supports you to engage positively with family, friends or colleagues, and deliver safe and compassionate care to your patients.

(RCN, 2024)

Self-care is the power we all hold as individuals to influence our well-being (Royal College of Nursing (RCN), 2024). In order to cultivate a number of self-care practices that will help you achieve balance in your life and enable you to focus on your well-being, the first step is to understand your values and beliefs, especially any self-limiting ones that might be holding you back from achieving your life and career goals. You might have a personal goal around fitness, which will make you more physically healthy, or perhaps a professional goal that a promotion will make you feel more powerful, and therefore a sign of being successful. However, once these things are achieved, we often then want something else to focus on. This motivational drive is often derived in childhood experiences and primary family relationships, or associated societal and culturally held expectations. It is important to learn how to realise what are assumptions and what are chosen values and beliefs, in order to set your mind free from any restrictions and limitations, instead opening your mind and attention to achieving what you want in life.

Study skills and a growth mindset

Developing a growth mindset is having belief that you can improve with effort. An expansive and open mind can help to approach challenges as opportunities rather than merely being seen as a threat or a setback.

REFLECTIVE LEARNING

From a study perspective, here are a number of self-care strategies that may be helpful.

SELF-CARE STRATEGIES

- Focus on time management and developing a study plan that will help manage coursework, practice hours, and personal life.
- Use planners, digital calendars, or productivity apps to help organise your diary effectively and reduce last-minute stress with assignment submissions, project deadlines, or practice assessments, for example.
- Setting realistic goals and breaking tasks into smaller manageable steps will help create a sense of accomplishment once completed.
- Schedule regular breaks to refresh your mind and manage stress more effectively.
- Allocate time for social activity, or a walk outside away from your desk, as something that brings you joy is important to build into your daily schedule no matter how long or short this might be; keeping things in balance is the key.
- Developing strong connections with fellow students and peers will help create an informal support system to enable you to share experiences, study in groups, and celebrate together.
- Finding a mentoring relationship, perhaps with academic tutors, clinical tutors, and practitioners on placement, will provide opportunity to seek advice and try out new ideas to help manage your time and life's stressors.
- Continuing to nurture relationships with friends and family helps keep you feeling connected and grounded, to seek support when you most need it, as well as have fun.
- Engaging in activities outside of your professional field, pursuing hobbies and interests.
- Participating in your local community perhaps through volunteering or activities that give back can bring a sense of purpose and connection with others, which in turn can enhance your personal happiness.
- Connecting with health professional communities such as student or national organisations helps to network and provides for additional support and inspiration, boosting your sense of belonging in your chosen professional field.

It is important to try and maintain your sense of purpose and remember your "why." Why you have come into the profession, why you are studying on your days off work, or why you care so much about what someone said, for example. Talking with your peers and mentor can assist your self-reflection so that you are aware of the bigger picture of what difference you can make in your role and foster a sense of achievement and interest in lifelong learning.

Reflective journalling

Keeping a reflective journal will help capture and process your thoughts, gain perspective, and help manage stress. It is helpful to write about challenges you have overcome, the insights learned, and the celebrations or positive moments you experienced along your journey. Reflective journalling also helps to regularly assess what matters most to you, personally and professionally.

I fill my own journal with things that have given me moments of joy, whether that be thank-you notes, photos, poems, pictures, as well as creating a reminder to myself of what I might do differently when I have experienced something that is in dissonance with my own values and has caused me stress. I use my own journal to hold reflective discussions with my personal coach. This helps to ensure I am celebrating achievements, no matter how small. I am also reflecting on how to make improvements so that the things I find stressful become a positive learning experience, giving me greater resources and a resilience to know what to do next time I experience something similar.

Journalling in this way also helps to focus on progress, rather than striving for ultimate perfection. When we make mistakes, or life gets tough, journalling can help becoming too self-critical. It can also help practice gratitude, which in turn helps to develop self-resilience.

Reflective exercise

- Use a reflective, creative journal to identify three positive things daily.
- What are the areas you feel you are falling short and need to address? Explore how.
- Celebrate small wins.
- Capture your mood in words, drawings, or artefacts (such as pictures, draw-ings, poems, cards, notes, etc.).
- Practice giving yourself a daily positive affirmation.
- Acknowledge progress made when addressing challenges, no matter how small.

- Develop habits that speak kindly to yourself, especially during difficult times. This in turn can help to manage self-doubt.

It is important to recognise that learning as a student is emotionally draining and that it is okay to feel stressed or anxious at times. Finding outlets to process your feelings in healthy ways is crucial, whether it be through talking to a trusted friend, mentor, or counsellor. Seeking mental health support when needed is not a sign of weakness; it is a strategy that will prove useful. Making contact through university counselling services or wellness programmes at your general practice (GP) will all help you to learn how manage stress throughout your life, so that things do not become overwhelming.

CONCLUSION

Health, wealth, and happiness are inextricably linked to well-being. Striving for balance is a lifelong mission. If you treat your body like it is the least important priority on your agenda, emotions will become more negative. This in turn will impair judgement, mental well-being, and work performance. Health and well-being affect relationships and engagement with the world around. Mind, body, and emotions are integrally linked, and one affects the other. By intentionally integrating self-care strategies into daily life, it is possible to create a more balanced approach to improve happiness, manage stress, and create a more fulfilling experience in both your personal and professional life.

FURTHER READING

The theoretical foundations for happiness

There are a large number of happiness frameworks designed for self-assessment that you can use to evaluate and improve your own personal well-being which focus on various dimensions of happiness and life satisfaction, helping you to identify areas for improving. Depending on your personal preferences and lifestyle, you can choose from the different frameworks identified in Table 1.1, and self-assessment tools in Table 1.2 subsequently, identify which resonates most, and go back to this resource as and when you or your teams need them.

Table 1.1 Self-assessment happiness frameworks.

Model/ framework name	Author	Elements measured	Self-assessment
PERMA model	Seligman (2011)	• Positive Emotions: Experiencing joy, pleasure, and contentment. • Engagement: Being deeply involved or absorbed in activities. • Relationships: Developing positive, meaningful connections with others. • Meaning: Finding purpose and significance in life. • Accomplishment: Achieving goals and feeling competent.	You can reflect on each of these dimensions by asking yourself how much of each you experience regularly. Online PERMA surveys are available to help quantify these elements and guide improvement
The Wheel of Life	Byrne (2005)	A popular coaching tool that allows individuals to assess different areas of their lives. Common dimensions include the following: • Career • Finances • Health • Relationships • Personal Growth • Recreation/Fun • Environment • Spirituality	You can rate your satisfaction in each of these areas on a scale (typically 1–10) and visualise them as spokes on a wheel. This tool helps identify imbalances and areas that may need more attention to achieve a sense of well-being. An example is provided in the final chapter.

(Continued)

Table 1.1 (Continued)

Model/framework name	Author	Elements measured	Self-assessment
The Happiness Index	Musikanski (2014)	Inspired by Bhutan's Gross National Happiness (GNH) and adapted for personal use, this tool assesses happiness across nine domains: • Psychological Well-being • Health • Education • Time Use • Cultural Diversity and Resilience • Good Governance • Community Vitality • Ecological Diversity and Resilience • Living Standards	Individuals can reflect on how each of these areas contributes to their overall happiness. Online tools like the "Happiness Index" offer structured questionnaires to rate well-being across these domains and track progress.
The Authentic Happiness Inventory (AHI)	Martin Seligman et al. (2005)	The AHI is a self-assessment tool that measures overall happiness and life satisfaction by asking a series of questions about positive emotions, life meaning, and personal accomplishment.	You can take the AHI online (available through the University of Pennsylvania's website) to receive a score that reflects your overall sense of happiness, along with suggestions for improvement.

(Continued)

Table 1.1 (Continued)

Model/ framework name	Author	Elements measured	Self-assessment
The Flourishing Scale	Ed Diener and Robert Biswas-Diener (2009)	Measures an individual's psychological well-being across several domains: • Relationships • Purpose • Self-acceptance • Mastery • Autonomy • Optimism	By scoring yourself on statements like "I lead a purposeful and meaningful life" and "I am optimistic about my future," you can get an overall measure of flourishing or thriving in life.
Satisfaction with Life Scale (SWLS)	Ed Diener et al. (1984)	SWLS measures life satisfaction through five simple statements, which participants rate on a scale from 1 to 7: • "In most ways, my life is close to my ideal." • "The conditions of my life are excellent." • "I am satisfied with my life." • "So far, I have gotten the important things I want in life." • "If I could live my life over, I would change almost nothing."	Individuals can quickly gauge their overall life satisfaction using this tool and compare their score to population averages.

(Continued)

Table 1.1 (Continued)

Model/ framework name	Author	Elements measured	Self-assessment
Ikigai framework	Sartore et al. (2023)	Originating from Japan, "Ikigai" refers to the concept of "reason for being." It encourages reflection across four overlapping dimensions: • What you love (Passion) • What you are good at (Profession) • What the world needs (Mission) • What you can be paid for (Vocation)	This framework helps explore what brings joy and fulfilment by identifying the sweet spot between these four areas. It's a useful tool for assessing purpose and meaning in life.
Gross National Happiness (GNH) Self-Assessment	Jigme Singye Wangchuck (1970s)	Although originally designed as a national framework by Bhutan, GNH principles can be adapted for personal use. It focuses on the balance of material, spiritual, and emotional well-being through the following domains: • Economic Wellness • Environmental Conservation • Good Governance • Cultural Preservation • Health and Education	Reflecting on how you score in these areas can provide insight into how various aspects of life contribute to your overall happiness.
The Oxford Happiness Questionnaire	Michael Argyle and Peter Hills	This questionnaire is a scientifically validated tool developed to measure personal happiness. It includes 29 questions that cover various aspects of well-being, including life satisfaction, self-esteem, and sense of purpose.	Individuals rate their responses to statements like "I feel that life is very rewarding" and "I am well satisfied about everything in my life." Results can indicate overall happiness and areas for improvement.

Table 1.2 Workplace tools and well-being approaches

Method	Description	Purpose
Self-assessment	Professional competence Self-assessment of your own competence and development needs which could include any professional framework that identifies the knowledge skills and know-how required to undertake your role effectively. e.g. RCN Principles of Nursing Practice www.rcn.org.uk/Professional-Development/Definition-and-principles-of-nursing Practice Assessment Record and Evaluation Tool (PARE) Self-assessment of your leadership at work using the Kouzes and Posner Leadership Practices Inventory (Kouzes and Posner 1993).	The principles describe what everyone, from nursing staff to people and populations, can expect from nursing to deliver safe and effective person-centred care. They cover the aspects of behaviour, attitude, and approach that underpin good care, and they are mapped to and complement the Nursing and Midwifery Council (NMC) Code (2024). Enables healthcare students to evaluate their placements and complete their practice assessment to meet the requirements of their professional regulator. Based on the Five Practices of Exemplary Leadership: 1. Model The Way 2. Inspire a Shared Vision 3. Challenge the Process 4. Enable Others to Act 5. Encourage the Heart Being a transformational and collective leader building relationships that encourage curiosity, creativity, and harnessing the talents of all, not just a few (Manley and Jackson 2020).

(Continued)

Table 1.2 (Continued)

Method	Description	Purpose
Qualitative 360-degree Feedback	This involves practitioners identifying their role and asking for open feedback from representatives of each role group in relation to four questions: • What is your understanding of my role? • What have you experienced that I do well in my role? • What constructive feedback can you give me to help me become more effective in my role? • What other feedback would you like to give me on my role?	• To develop role clarity for self and others. • To begin to learn how to give and receive open and direct feedback about one's effectiveness. • To develop skills in qualitative analysis of data. The first two characteristics (role clarity and giving and receiving feedback) are essential for effective workplace cultures.
Reflective Review	This method, based on the work of Chris Johns (1995), encourages participants to reflect on their experience of actively learning together with a group by using the following reflective questions: • What are your aims and hopes at the beginning of your active learning? • What internal and external factors will help or hinder you in the process of active learning? • What are the main work themes that emerge for you? • What is your learning from the process? • What are the work themes that you need to address for the future?	Encourages participants to link their past and present learning to their future ways of working by encouraging them to reflect on their experience in active learning sets and in using the reflective review methods.

REFERENCES

Byrne, U. (2005) Wheel of Life: Effective Steps For Stress Management. *Business Information Review*, 22(2):123–130.

Diener, E. (1984) Subjective well-being. *Psychological bulletin*, 95(3):542.

Diener, E. and Ryan, K. (2009) Subjective well-being: A general overview. *South African journal of psychology*, 39(4):391–406.

Finney L. (2013) *Our Shared Purpose: A Practical Guide*. Horsham, UK: Roffey Park Institute.

Gerodimos V., Karatrantou K., Papazeti K., Batatolis C. and Krommidas C. (2022) Workplace exercise program in a hospital environment: An effective strategy for the promotion of employees physical and mental health. A randomized controlled study. *International Archives of Environmental Occupational Health*. 95:1491–1500. https://doi.org/10.1007/s00420-022-01856-6.

Ghahramani S., Kasraei H., Hayati R., Tabrizi R. and Marzaleh M.A. (2023) Health care workers' mental health in the face of COVID-19: A systematic review and meta-analysis. *International Journal of Psychiatry Clinical Practice*. 27:208–217. https://doi.org/10.1080/13651501.2022.2101927.

Hill J.E., Harris C., Danielle L.C., Boland P., Doherty A.J., Benedetto V., Gita B.E. and Clegg A.J. (2022) The prevalence of mental health conditions in healthcare workers during and after a pandemic: Systematic review and meta-analysis. *Journal of Advanced Nursing*. 78:1551–1573. https://doi.org/10.1111/jan.15175.

Jakobsen M.D., Sundstrup E., Brandt M., Jay K., Aagaard P. and Andersen L.L. (2015) Effect of workplace- versus home-based physical exercise on musculoskeletal pain among healthcare workers: A cluster randomized controlled trial. *Scandinavian Journal Work Environment Health*. 41:153–163. https://doi.org/10.5271/sjweh.3479.

Kouzes J.M. and Posner B.Z. (1993) *Leadership Practices Inventory. A Self-assessment and Analysis*, expanded ed., San Francisco, CA: Jossey-Bass.

Li Y., Scherer N., Felix L. and Kuper H. (2021) Prevalence of depression, anxiety and post-traumatic stress disorder in health care workers during the COVID-19 pandemic: A systematic review and meta-analysis. *PLoS ONE*. 16:e0246454. https://doi.org/10.1371/journal.pone.0246454.

Lomas T., Medina J.C., Ivtzan I., Rupprecht S. and Eiroa-Orosa F.J. (2018) A systematic review of the impact of mindfulness on the well-being of healthcare professionals. *Journal of Clinical Psychology*. 74:319–355. https://doi.org/10.1002/jclp.22515.

Manley K. and Jackson C. (2020) The Venus model for integrating practitioner-led workforce transformation and complex change across the health care system. *Journal of Evaluation in Clinical Practice*. 26:622–634.

Manley K., O'Keefe H., Jackson C. Pearce J. and Smith S. (2014) A shared purpose framework to deliver person-centred safe and effective care: Organisational transformation using practice development methodology. *International Journal of Practice Development*. 4. Article 2. https://doi.org/10.19043/ipdj.41.002.

Manley K., O'Keefe H. and Jackson C. (2011a) *Providing Person-centred, Safe and Effective Care: A Framework for East Kent University NHS Foundation Trust: The Contribution of Nursing and Midwifery Practice and Clinical Leadership*. Final Report Unpublished. Revised Final Report, Published 2014. Canterbury, UK: England Centre for Practice Development.

Manley K., Sanders K., Cardiff S. and Webster J. (2011b) Effective workplace culture: the attributes, enabling factors and consequences of a new concept. *International Practice Development Journal*. 1(2):1–29.

McCormack, B. and McCance, T. eds. (2017) *Person-Centred Practice in Nursing and Health Care: Theory and Practice*. Oxford: John Wiley and Sons.

Müller A., Heiden B., Herbig B., Poppe F. and Angerer P. (2016) Improving well-being at work: A randomized controlled intervention based on selection, optimization, and compensation. *Journal of Occupational Health Psychology*. 21:169–181. https://doi.org/10.1037/a0039676.

Musikanski, L. (2014) Happiness in public policy. *Journal of Sustainable Social Change*, 6(1):5.

Perez G.K., Haime V., Jackson V., Chittenden E., Mehta D.H. and Park E.R. (2017) Promoting resiliency among palliative care clinicians: Stressors, coping strategies, and training needs. *Journal of Palliative Medicine*. 18:332–337.

Romero-Sanchez J.M., Porcel-Galvez A.M., Paloma-Castro O., Garcia-Jimenez J., Gonzalez-Dominguez M.E., Palomar-Aumatell X. and Fernandez-Garcia E. (2022) Worldwide prevalence of inadequate work ability among hospital nursing personnel: A systematic review and meta-analysis. *Journal of Nursing Scholarship*. 54:513–528. doi: 10.1111/jnu.12749.

Royal College of Nursing (2024) *Definition and Principles of Nursing*. www.rcn.org.uk/Professional-Development/Definition-and-principles-of-nursing

Sartore, M., Buisine, S., Ocnarescu, I. and Joly, L. R. (2023) An integrated cognitive-motivational model of ikigai (purpose in life) in the workplace. *Europe's Journal of Psychology*. 19(4):387.

Seligman, M. E. (2011) Building resilience. *Harvard business review*. 89(4):100–106.

Seligman, M. E. P., Steen, T. A., Park, N. and Peterson, C. (2005) Positive psychology progress: Empirical validation of interventions. *American Psychologist*, 60:410–421.doi:10.1037/0003-066X.60.5.410

Sheldon G.F., Ricketts T.C., Charles A., King J., Fraher E.P. and Meyer A. (2008) The global health workforce shortage: Role of surgeons and other providers. *Advances in Surgery*. 42:63–85. https://doi.org/10.1016/j.yasu.2008.04.006

Shiri R. Nikunlaakso R. and Laitinen J. (2023) Effectiveness of workplace interventions to improve health and well-being of health and social service workers: A narrative review of randomised controlled trials. *Healthcare* (Basel). 11(12):1792. https://doi.org/10.3390/healthcare11121792. PMID: 37372909; PMCID: PMC10298158.

Spinelli C., Wisener M. and Khoury B. (2019) Mindfulness training for healthcare professionals and trainees: A meta-analysis of randomized controlled trials. *Journal of Psychometric Research*. 120:29–38. https://doi.org/10.1016/j.jpsychores.2019.03.003.

Steptoe A., Deaton A.M. and Stone A.A. (2015) Subjective wellbeing, health and ageing. *Lancet*. 385:640–48.

Steptoe A. (2019) Happiness and Health. *Annual Review of Public Health*. 40:339–59.

Taylor H., Cavanagh K., Field A.P. and Strauss C. (2022) Health care workers' need for headspace: Findings from a multisite definitive randomized controlled trial of an unguided digital mindfulness-based self-help app to reduce healthcare worker stress. *JMIR mHealth uHealth*.10:e31744. https://doi.org/10.2196/31744.

United Nations (2019) World Happiness Report. Available via https://www.worldhappiness.report/ed/2019/ (last accessed 6/10/2025).

van Dijk I., Lucassen P., Akkermans R.P., van Engelen B.G.M., van Weel C. and Speckens A.E.M. (2017) Effects of mindfulness-based stress reduction on the mental health of clinical clerkship students: A cluster-randomized controlled trial. *Journal of the Association of the American Medical* Colleges. 92:1012–1021. https://doi.org/10.1097/ACM.0000000000001546.

Waldinger R. and Shculzm, M. (2023) *The Good Life: Lessons from the World's Longest Scientific Study of Happiness*. New York, NY: Simon and Schuster Inc.

World Health Organization (1948) Summary Reports on Proceedings Minutes and Final Acts of the International Health Conference held in New York from 19 June to 22 July 1946. World Health Organization, available from: https://apps.who.int/iris/handle/10665/85573.

Chapter 2
Survival of the workforce

Oscar Noel Ocho

INTRODUCTION

Global health systems are mostly developed to meet the needs of population health through offering services at different levels of prevention, extending from primary to secondary and tertiary levels of care provision. Effective leadership is identified as key to the effectiveness of all the different levels of health and care systems. Yet globally there are systemic challenges that even the most effective approach to leadership within contemporary and changing models of integrated health and care systems can impact on a person's effectiveness. Lartey Sarah et al., (2023) argued that health systems have become increasingly more complex, and as a result, this requires a vast and transferable skill set, if leaders are to become and remain successful in their workplace.

SELF-EFFICACY IN LEADERSHIP WITHIN CONTEMPORARY HEALTH SYSTEMS

Self-efficacy has emerged as an important concept in leadership development. Data has shown a significant impact on 'readiness' as well as 'effectiveness' in assuming leadership roles within organizations Lartey Sarah et al. (2023). However, Dwyer (2019) argues that although system level adaptability is identified as an effective strategy for successful leadership, as a construct itself, self-efficacy has significant variability in definition, development and measurement of these associated constructs. While there is some level of emphasis on behaviours associated with effective leadership, new and emerging literature shows that contemporary health systems must extend beyond leadership as the individual's personal traits, moving more to an emphasis on corporate and consistent group behaviours. Exacerbated by the dynamics associated with the work environment, emerging leadership focuses is on the development of leadership as an organizational skill and not just a focus on an individual's personal attributes and status of any one selected individual Dubey, Pathak and Sahu, (2023).

DOI: 10.4324/9781041057956-3

CASE STUDY

Joan has been a qualified registered nurse (RN) for the last ten years. She is very assertive and has invested much time in preparing herself for the position of ward manager. She has gained further qualifications, achieving several courses and is in the final stages of completing a master's degree, with an emphasis on health leadership and administration. She is one of the most qualified nurses on the ward and carries herself with a sense of superiority over her colleagues. Although she is very knowledgeable, others have observed a challenge with her clinical practice. She has not been able to demonstrate clinical competence in practice, as she gets others to execute her practical assignments by giving them personal favors. However, Joan is an extremely proficient nurse who has extensive years of experience in the clinical area. Joan says she likes 'bedside nursing' but has no desire to do any further clinical-based studies.

Matron Steff has informed you that the position of ward manager will be advertised internally and that she is keen to have a reference from you, as the ward's clinical supervisor, so that they can apply, as it is a permanent position, whereas the matron role is only interim. You have an excellent working relationship with both matron and with Joan, and believe that both of them are eligible for the position. However, some members of staff have told you privately that if either person is recommended for the position, they would ask for a reassignment since they are of the view that both persons are not suitably qualified or clinically able to deal with such a position, based on prior experience or their qualifications. Nevertheless, the service has been highlighted as one of the best functioning units within the organization, which has brought much recognition by the executive team, and you are often featured in the newsletters and on social media for work being achieved.

Meanwhile, Joan has been attempting to gather supporters from staff, as she is of the view that she is best positioned based on her level of qualifications. Her pitch is that she will be able to bring some of the more current theoretical principles of leadership to bear on her position. She is of the view that based on her observations, she is well-positioned to make a big difference as a leader, since clinical competence should not be given priority over academic preparation. Such 'peacock' behaviour is affecting staff, who express to you they are feeling as though clinical skills are somehow less valued than academic qualifications, and they keep wanting to get supervision time with you to discuss where and how they might be better suited to build a career elsewhere.

CRITICAL QUESTIONS FOR CONSIDERATION

1. What is the problem in this scenario?
2. If you were the ward clinical supervisor, what are some of the self-efficacy issues that you might need to consider in informing your recommendation for the role of ward manager?
3. If you were in Joan's position, what are some of the personal or professional considerations that you would need to consider in determining your readiness for the position and how this might impact on the team functioning and ward's reputation?
4. What are some of the actions that you would consider in supporting both members of staff, in how you might be able to support their self-efficacy, readiness and preparation for the application, interview and potentially the subsequent ward manager position?

LEADERSHIP SELF-EFFICACY

Leadership self-efficacy has been defined as 'an estimate of one's ability to successfully execute the behavior required to produce desired outcomes' (Dwyer, 2019 p637). While this definition focuses on the individual's perception of competence, this also requires examination of the context (i.e. organization) and complexity of associated health systems alongside theoretical principles that affects leaders' behaviors within specific contexts. This is particularly important since every organization, no matter how much emphasis it may place on the importance of developing shared values and ownership, comprises individuals who are more heterogenous than homogenous. In other words, any organization is made up of the people who work there, as they are central to how that organization functions.

The role of self-efficacy in leadership development has been recognized as more complex than traditionally considered (Machida and Schaubroeck, 2011). Health care settings are complex contexts, where leadership behaviours are considered critical to organizational success. For example, leadership behaviours may be considered appropriate and effective in one particular organization, but may be viewed differently when applied within other contexts. How variations in leadership behaviours are measured will therefore be systematically difficult to measure, as there is a dependence on the application of principles of leadership rather than a 'lift and shift' concrete approach. This variability has been identified as one of the limitations in measuring self-efficacy, as there is a potential to pay little attention to the contextual factors that affect leadership behaviours and self-efficacy (Dwyer, 2019).

In this chapter, leadership self-efficacy is defined as *the aptitudes, attitudes and competencies of leaders to navigate the leadership challenges within the workplace environment*. As a consequence, the emphasis will not be on how self-efficacy affects leadership success, but more about influencing the individual's capacity to function optimally in a complex and ever-changing environment.

Machida and Schaubroeck (2011) state that self-efficacy beliefs are central to leadership development. They argued that leader self-efficacy is different to leadership self-efficacy, as the leader operates at the level of the individual, but leadership is more focused on the impacts of working with or leading a group. In can be inferred then that how an individual perceives themselves, in relation to the leadership role, will have a critical influence on their understanding of their core competencies and/or deficiencies, which can influence their capacity to function optimally. Whilst emphasis on leadership self-efficacy is not about leadership styles (of the individual leader), there has been greater emphasis on how leader self-efficacy contributes to the emergence and development of leaders within organizations (Bergman, Gustafsson-Sendén and Berntson, 2021; Bobbio and Manganelli, 2009; Bracht et al., 2021; Krampitz et al., 2021; Machida and Schaubroeck, 2011).

Although there is evidence that leader self-efficacy has been associated with leadership success and favourable work outcomes (Bobbio and Manganelli, 2009; Bracht et al., 2021; Dwyer, 2019; Machida and Schaubroeck, 2011), consideration must be given to the socio-cultural environment in which leaders emerge (Bracht et al., 2021).

Bracht et al., (2021) argued that a leader's characteristics can have a positive influence on the followers' characteristics within the work environment, since emphasis is to increase team functioning rather than merely emphasize the position of the leader. However, there is some level of ambiguity in the literature since self-efficacy focuses on the leader's beliefs about their own competence, which may be more associated with how the leaders assert themselves in the workplace. Yet, impact of the leaders' performance in terms of how a leader performs within the organization, especially those fraught with complexities, may extend beyond self-perception, and has more to do with consistency of actions in the position of being a leader, as witnessed and experiences by those who follow (Bergman, Gustafsson-Sendén and Berntson, 2021). When leadership exists within a team context of 'followers', whatever the configuration, effectiveness must be measured from the perspective of the one who is in the position of authority, as well as from those who operate within the organizational context as the 'followers'.

Leader self-efficacy, then, focuses on utilizing one's belief in personal competence to work with teams towards the achievement of a common goal in such a way that it would impact positively on the organization's outcomes (Bergman, Gustafsson-Sendén and Berntson, 2021).

Lee (1989) argued that while self-efficacy theory has been widely accepted in the literature, the theory does not go far enough in explaining human behaviour, which makes the theoretical explanation illusionary. Krampitz et al., (2021), in conducting a meta-analysis, found that self-leadership influenced how leaders perceived their self-efficacy, which impacted on their performance. As a consequence, if the arguments about self-efficacy are focused on leader success, this may be challenging, since consideration has to be given to the nuances as well as the socio-cultural milieu in which the leader operates.

EXAMINING THE MULTIDIMENSIONAL CONCEPT OF LEADERSHIP

As with previous discussion on a leader's self-efficacy, the concept of leadership itself is associated with navigating between the characteristics of the leader, alongside the context in which the leader has to operate.

There are a number of factors that affect leadership effectiveness identified in the vast amounts of literature available. Table 2.1 below has captured some of these to reveal the balance between the individual, their context and opportunities available.

While there are some identified core constructs about successful leaders that are supported in the literature, leadership remains a dynamic concept and requires constant review. As can be seen from the table earlier, it is important that any leader needs to remain open to new learning and opportunities, particularly if leaders are to remain contemporary, flexible, adaptive to the context and highly effective (Machida and Schaubroeck, 2011).

Several models and frameworks for effective leadership have been developed over the years, which moved from focusing on the personal traits of the leader to a shared ownership approach to leadership, looking at what occurs between

Table 2.1 Factors affecting leadership potentials

Individual	Context	Opportunities
• reluctance to change • lack of vision and commitment • lack of system level awareness, particularly how to lead at the higher system levels • lack of incentives • loss of confidence (arising from previous or past experiences) • inadequate communication • role conflict • lack of recognition and influence • time constraints to pursue leadership development	• poor teamwork • lack of vision and commitment • lack of incentives • interdisciplinary relationships • preparation for leadership roles • role conflict • perceived need for further leadership development	• lack of incentives • limited organizational leadership opportunities • lack of funding for advancement as a leader, • interdisciplinary relationships • constant reconfiguration of service structures

Source: created by Oscar Noel Ocho.

the leaders and their subordinates (Day David et al, 2014). Identified nuances and challenges associated with conceptualization of leadership development versus the leaders own development, which are dynamic and associated with individual, as well as corporate characteristics. Bush, Michalek and Francis, (2020) argued that while leadership style was associated with leadership outcomes, this did not translate into perceptions of leadership self-efficacy.

Hoang, Luu and Yang, (2025) explored authentic leadership in the tourism sector. They stated that leadership was critical in such a sector because of the general public's demands for quality, tailored experience and a responsive service. The health care system is perhaps no different. Like the tourism sector, the health sector is fraught with uncertainties and persistent change. Modern health care is contending with a more litigious conscious clientele who have expectations of what they require, are researching their ailments and comparing service offers via the internet, as well as having high expectations of what will be accepted as a quality service experience.

Attributes for authentic leadership

Authentic leadership has a focus on the personal attributes of the leader who is responsible for providing leadership. An authentic leader remains reflective of their principles, which are to be aligned with a values-based approach to leadership, as well as remaining aware of context through, for example, mapping their activities to organizational priorities.

Hoang, Luu and Yang, (2025) argued that authentic leadership has been shown to be more effective than transformational and ethical leadership, although transformational leadership has been well-established and supported in the literature (Bush, Michalek and Francis, 2020). In such circumstances, authentic leaders need to ensure their behaviours are aligned to principles of equity, consistency, openness and transparency, which in turn must be consistent and align well with the organization's vision and mission.

There is some consensus on the importance of key attributes to leadership success within organizations (Algunmeeyn et al., 2023; Gutterman, 2023; Hargett et al., 2017). Some of the key attributes for effective leadership have been recognized as

- approachability, effective communication and clinical skills, honesty, integrity, support for others and visibility (Algunmeeyn et al., 2023); and
- integrity, effective communication, adherence to ethical values, building relationships and critical thinking (Hargett et al., 2017).

Complexity and professional work environment

Vickie Hughes (2018) conducted a comprehensive review of the literature on the barriers to effective leadership. These include inadequate levels of preparation, the changing leadership structures, as well as constant reconfiguration of health systems, career path trajectory and motivations to position oneself in leadership as well as absence of succession planning. (Refer again to Table 2.1 earlier.)

These factors are critical in contexts where there is low level of human and material resources which may be more pronounced in small and developing island states (SDIs), and in government funded organizations effected by global economy downturn. What is even more critical is the reality that SDIs experience, in an exacerbation of their human resource challenges by having to contend with the perennial challenges associated with staff migration. As a consequence, there is a level of dependence on younger, inexperienced practitioners, who will be expected to assume and function effectively as leaders, yet with inadequate levels of preparation (Ocho et al., 2020b). What is even more challenging is the observation that health systems are more focused on replacement planning (recruitment) rather than succession (retainment and retention) planning (Gabriel, Biriowu and Dagogo, 2020; Ocho et al., 2020a, 2020b). While Gabriel, Biriowu and Dagogo (2020) argued that both strategies are important, replacement planning is often used for short-term approach to filling vacancies, whilst strategic workforce planning focuses on a more longer-term approach to human resource management, future service redesigns and therefore an associated need for evidence-based workforce modelling.

While strategic workforce planning may be considered most plausible for effective systems management, this may not be possible in situations where staff migration continues to drain the available skilled and experienced staff. In some instances, managers are unable to adequately implement strategies for succession planning, or service improvements, since remaining staff may need to proceed on vacation leave, only to then correspond with their administrative teams towards the end of their leave stating that they would be resigning their positions. This is particularly challenging for managers as they have to rely on replacement planning in the short to medium term, to secure a level of safe staffing, whilst giving consideration to effective recruitment from a strategic planning perspective.

WORKFORCE CHALLENGES

Workforce challenges are further exacerbated by problems in circumstances where the person who was replaced may not necessarily be the most suitable, experienced or prepared and may not necessarily be employed, or promoted substantively into the position (refer again to the case study). In such situations, there is often a disconnect between personal and organizational expectation that has potential to affect staff morale and their commitment to the organization. While there is often a tendency to have vacancies filled quickly, even when considering replacement planning (Gabriel, Biriowu and Dagogo, 2020), this may not necessarily improve organizational effectiveness, as considerations may not be given to the 'most suitable' candidate. Consequently, leaders within organizations will have to consider what may be the most plausible action to be taken in the short to medium term, to facilitate organizational continuity rather than overall performance effectiveness.

Another challenge within the organization context is expectations between workers representing different chronological groups, such as Generation X (those born from 1965 to 1980) and Generation Z (those born from 1997 to 2012). While staff associated with both generations belong to multiple professions within health systems, their perceptions of their role, commitment to a shared organizational vision or career trajectory may be very different.

Jujuk and Tridayanti, (2024) who argued that not only are the styles of leadership different but the technological and intellectual environment within which generations operate are different. As a consequence, organizations are expected to be able to embrace new workplace practices, embrace flexible working, enhanced use of technologies, which represents different demographics, as well as impacting the required approaches to leadership including a move to a more dispersive leadership style, including introducing democratic engagement of staff through shared governance, for example.

IMPLICATIONS FOR SELF-EFFICACY IN LEADERSHIP

From a conceptual level, there is some level of ambivalence in the literature on how self-efficacy is to be measured as it has to be juxtaposed to the types of behaviours exhibited in specific contexts (Lee, 1989; Krampitz et al., 2021). There are five key self-efficacy factors that should be considered that will be useful to support your effectiveness as a leaders, and your self-efficacy, as the aptitude, attitudes and behaviours of collective leaders if they are to function optimally in complex organizations.

1: Being authentic

Being authentic will necessitate that an individual comes into the position of leadership with the requisite technical, personal and academic competence required for navigating the organizational landscape, whilst aligning these to their personal values and beliefs. No matter the size or dynamics that exist within an organization, there is need for leaders to set clear and realistic goals, setting a shared vision as well as provide strategic leadership within the organization. Sometimes, there is conflict between how a person perceives themselves, as opposed to what is actually required to operate with a level of proficiency in the position of leadership, within that organizational structure and workplace culture. One of the key attributes required amongst aspiring leaders is authenticity.

Within organizations, team members want to know their leaders possess the requisite technical academic and professional competence to execute the requirements of the job. While there may be opportunities provided for understanding unique challenges that are context specific, there will be no such consideration if the members of the team recognize that the leader is not authentic.

While Gardner William et al. (2021) argue that the concept of authentic leadership is in itself fraught with many challenges, including conceptual and methodological challenges, there is some level of consensus of its importance in practice. Nevertheless, one cannot underestimate the importance of ensuring that within any organization, a leader must be true to their ideals and demonstrate the same level of consistency, in spite of the changing context in which they operate. This will be deemed necessary as organizations are fluid entities which allow for throughput amongst personnel who may be observing through interactions with their leaders, whether there is consistency of action as well as competence to function in different circumstances. This perspective was supported by Datta (2015) who postulated that a leader's effectiveness is measured by the workers' or other outside stakeholders' perceptions of the leader to maintain team effectiveness.

Alilyyani, Wong and Cummings (2018), in conducting a systematic review on antecedents, mediators and outcomes of authentic leadership in health care, found that authentic leadership had positive outcomes from two perspectives, the health care team, and ultimately on patient outcomes.

Authentic leadership was relational in nature as members of staff are able to observe the behaviour of the leader, which contributes to building trust and respect amongst members of the team. This is particularly important in complex organizations where there is competition for recognition, space at the table, as a powerful leverage for decision making within the organization. A leader who is not seen as being authentic may be more likely to have their leadership position questioned. Being authentic will require adopting a position of being ethical in decision making and demonstrating equity in how relations with staff are established.

2. **Balancing expectations**

One of the key areas to be considered in managing expectations amongst leaders is to remain open to the need for a change (Rahayu and Tridayanti, 2024). They argued that leadership styles affect staff motivation depending on generational age. What can be challenging for some leaders is contending with generational differences that could place additional burdens on their adopted leadership approach, and draw upon their self-efficacy to cope appropriately to accommodate these. This has been highlighted in the changing workplace environment, especially in the post COVID-19 era, where new approaches to workplace efficiency have quickly been adopted, including working in an online environment, with reduced available hours together spent in the physical workplace environment, persistent budget and resource constraints imposed, with even greater reliance on Artificial Intelligence (AI) to facilitate administrative, routine and daily activities.

Individuals come to work bringing different levels of expertise. As a leader with effective self-efficacy skills, one is able to recognize the importance of validating the contributions of all members of the team, based on their level of expertise, areas of interest and talents, promoting leadership attributes amongst all the team members. This validating approach has the potential of boosting camaraderie and effective workplace interactions since it is based on a deliberate balancing of expectations between the role of the leader and a recognition of expertise from amongst colleagues in the workplace.

Jafarinia et al. (2019) achieved a meta synthesis to support this position when they argued that the younger generation come into the workplace looking for opportunities for personal and professional development and that it is incumbent on leaders to validate their ambitions and concerns by developing strategies to retain them in the organizations. This assumes importance in contexts where the millennials are looking for job marketability as opposed to job security, since the workplace can be viewed as a transient stop on the trajectory to economic freedom. In such circumstances, the younger workforce generations may be more inclined to position themselves to achieve whatever brings success, as patchwork careers, rather than feel aligned to the organization, or indeed just one chosen profession. In these circumstances, leaders must develop a level of sensitivity to the fact that expectations as well as outcomes will differ and it has nothing to do with questioning the authority or legitimacy of the leader.

3. Taking time for self-care

Research has shown that leaders who pay attention to self-care activities are more effective as leaders (Klug, Felfe and Krick, 2022). They further argued that health-oriented leadership is predicated on two assumptions; the first is that self-caring leaders are more willing and able to provide care for staff care; and second, leaders act as role models for their employees, which inspires others to engage in self-care.

Work demands can become overwhelming, often exacerbated by having to meet deadlines, manage personnel and align budgets, all within limited or restricted resources. Such situations pose significant challenges for leaders, especially if they feel anxious about how they may be failing their employees, colleagues and/or patients. Such leaders may find themselves having to navigate the demands of their jobs with their personal responsibility for caring for their families, let alone themselves – a challenge that we all know well enough can be extremely demanding. Nevertheless, research has shown that leaders who model effective self-care have a positive effect on their subordinates and their own self-care as well (Klug, Felfe and Krick, 2022).

The importance of leaders taking time for self-care has become more pronounced in the post COVID-19 era. The very nature of the job, as the helping profession, poses cognitive dissonance for many health care professionals, especially if they perceive that time out of being busy at work for self-care can result in harm somehow arising to staff as well as the clients whom they serve. Urick, Carpenter and Eckert (2021) argue that since health care is an essential service there is an increased likelihood of burnout, as well as role strain, which can be equally challenging for staff. In this regard, many leaders have to confront the importance of mentoring and coaching their staff while having to deal with very personal fears and challenges (Ocho et al., 2020b).

While accountability lies with the leader, there is a commensurate level of personal responsibility for leaders to take time to care for themselves. What this requires is that leaders adopt a space, whether mental or physical, that is considered almost sacred, which will allow them opportunities for uninterrupted reflection, relaxation and reinvigoration. Such a space and time should be respected by members of the team for it is the modeling of such personal 'time-out' activities that are likely to motivate others to adopt self-care as a key strategy in addressing workplace stressors.

REFLECTIVE ACTIVITY

Reflect on your scores for the items in each domain of your personal self-care audit tool.

DEVELOPING A SELF-CARE PLAN

1. List the self-care habits you are using now to manage stress and stay healthy.
2. List the self-care habits you would like to use but are not currently practising.
3. Identify the obstacles keeping you from practising these habits.
4. What solutions can you come up with to address the obstacles you listed?
5. For the self-care habits you wrote down for item 2, select one you would like to begin practising and complete the subsequent sentences:

Today I commit to
_____

I want to do this because
_____

I will accomplish this by
_____

Figure 2.1 Developing a Self-Care Plan: Khan, 2022 (unpublished/open source)

4. Self-confidence

Leaders, by the very nature of their functions, will be responsible for representing their staff and patient populations at different levels of management within and sometimes external to their employing organizations. Leaders will often be required to make representation through the articulation of a well-crafted business case, or represent staff on board meetings, in responsible positions addressing issues that affect the workforce. In a high-intensity and complex organization there is a tendency to consider individual needs, while, at the same time, senior management expects a level of systems thinking, which may require making compromise or allowing other priorities to supersede their own immediate concerns based on other pressures. In such situations leaders must be resilient enough to decipher the difference between understanding the importance of alignment of one's own interests with that of the organization, as opposed to believing that they, or their team, are being attacked personally.

Having a sense of self-confidence will go a long way in ensuring that such leaders will be able to articulate their point of view assertively, and with a sense of self-confidence, with the potential to persuade other stakeholders to listen and respond to what is being asked.

Kane et al. (2021), in conducting a systematic review, found that self-confidence is the basis for developing human agency that sets the framework for self-efficacy. However, findings from the review showed that there was some level of ambivalence since there was difficulty in making conclusions about the effect of self-confidence and its impact on self-efficacy since the constructs could not have been effectively measured.

Reflective task

Rate the following areas by frequency as they currently apply to your life.

Personal self-care audit tool

5 = Frequently, 4 = Occasionally, 3 = Rarely, 2 = Never, 1 = It never occurred to me

You can use the ratings to identify areas you may want to give more focus to.

Table 2.2 Self-assessment tool adapted from Saakvitne, K. W., & Pearlman, L. A. (1996)

Domain	Rating
Physical self-care	
Eat regularly (e.g., breakfast, lunch, dinner)	
Eat healthily	
Exercise (at least 30 mins a day, 5 days a week)	
Get regular medical care for prevention	
Get medical care when needed	
Take time off when sick	
Get massages	
Dance, swim, walk, run, play sports, sing, or do some other physical activity that is fun	
Take time to be sexual with self or with partner	
Get enough sleep	
Wear clothes you like	
Take vacations	
Take day trips or mini vacations	
Make time away from telephones or screens	
Other: _____	
Psychological self-care	
Make time for self-reflection	

(Continued)

Table 2.2 (Continued)

Domain	Rating
Have your own personal psychotherapy	
Write in a journal	
Read literature that is unrelated to your work	
Do something at which you are not an expert or in charge	
Decrease stress in your life	
Notice your inner experience – listen to your thoughts, judgements, beliefs, attitudes and feelings	
Let others know different aspects of you	
Engage your intelligence in a new area; e.g., go to an art museum, sports event, theatre performance	
Practise receiving from others	
Be curious	
Say no to extra responsibilities	
Other: _____	
Emotional self-care	
Spend time with others whose company you enjoy	
Stay in contact with important people in your life	
Give yourself affirmations, praise yourself	
Love yourself	
We read favourite books, re-watch favourite movies	
Identify comforting activities, objects, people, relationships, places and seek them out	
Allow yourself to cry	
Find things that make you laugh	

(Continued)

Table 2.2 (Continued)

Domain	Rating
Express your passion in social action, letters, donations, activism	
Play with children	
Other: _____	
Spiritual self-care	
Make time for reflection	
Spend time with nature	
Find a spiritual connection or community	
Be open to inspiration	
Cherish your optimism and hope	
Be aware of nonmaterial aspects of life	
Try at times not to be in charge or the expert	
Be open to not knowing	
Identify what is meaningful to you and notice its place in your life	
Meditate	
Pray	
Sing	
Spend time with children	
Have experiences of awe	
Contribute to causes in which you believe	
Read inspirational literature (listen to talks, music, etc.)	
Other: _____	
Workplace or professional self-care	
Take a break during the workday (e.g., lunch)	

(Continued)

Table 2.2 (Continued)

Domain	Rating
Take time to chat with co-workers	
Make quiet time to complete tasks	
Identify projects or tasks that are exciting and rewarding	
Set limits with clients and colleagues	
Balance your caseload so no one day or part of the day is too much	
Arrange your workspace so it is comfortable and comforting	
Get regular supervision or consultation	
Negotiate for your needs (benefits, pay raise)	
Have a peer support group	
Develop an area of professional interest outside your specialization	
Other: _____	
Other areas of self-care that are important or relevant to you	
Other: _____	
Other: _____	
Other: _____	

5. Building supportive networks

Leading teams and leadership can be very lonely for many leaders. Especially if they are new to the leadership team, or there are not many other roles of a similar level in their organization to seek out peers. One of the key lessons that effective leaders need to learn is the importance of building strong networks with stakeholders internal and external to the organization.

Research has shown that building strong social and professional networks supports self-efficacy within organizations (Bjorklund et al., 2020; Liou and Daly, 2020; Siciliano, 2016). Siciliano (2016) argued that when networks are considered, it is not the quantity but the quality of the networks that have been shown to be effective in building self-efficacy as a leader. Leaders should take care in building networks, as it will necessitate making oneself vulnerable with other stakeholders. Consequently, this will require trust and the development of shared interests while at the same time maintaining one's authenticity as a leader. The major challenge in this regard will be to ensure that the leader does not lose his individuality while ensuring alignment with others whom he/she perceives as being important to their networks.

CONCLUSION

Throughout this chapter, focus has been on developing an understanding of self-efficacy within the complicated workplace context of health and social care. Yet the literature tells us a lot about how to improve self-efficacy, through a series of attributes, behaviours and awareness. Dealing with the challenges of complicated systems and workforce challenges has been explored. Through remaining open to the situation, and adapting leadership style to the context, remaining open to change and lifelong learning is the key to a long and successful career as a leader. Taking time for self-care remains a core element to being and role modelling authentic leadership practices. All the best in your chosen approach to being and remaining true to you, as an authentic and highly effective leader – no matter where you work or where you are on your chosen career ladder.

REFERENCES

Algunmeeyn, A., Mrayyan, M.T., Suliman, W.A., Abunab, H.Y. and Al-Rjoub, S.F. (2023) Effective clinical nursing leadership in hospitals: Barriers from the perspectives of nurse managers. *BMJ Leader*, 8, 20–24

Alilyyani Bayan, Wong Carol A. and Cummings Greta. (2018) Antecedents, mediators, and outcomes of authentic leadership in healthcare: A systematic review. *International Journal of Nursing Studies*, 83, 34–64. ISSN 0020–7489. https://doi.org/10.1016/j.ijnurstu.2018.04.001.

Bergman, D., Gustafsson-Sendén, M. and Berntson, E (2021) From believing to doing: The association between leadership self-efficacy and the developmental leadership. *Model. Front. Psychol.* 12, 669905. https://doi.org/10.3389/fpsyg.2021.669905

Bjorklund, P., Daly, A. J., Ambrose, R. and van Es, E. A. (2020) Connections and capacity: An exploration of preservice teachers' sense of belonging, social networks, and self-efficacy in three teacher education programs. *AERA Open*. 6(1), https://doi.org/10.1177/2332858420901496

Bobbio, A. and Manganelli, A. M. (2009) Multidimensional leadership self-efficacy scale: A new multidimensional instrument. *Testing, Psychometrics, Methodology in Applied Psychology.* 16(1), 3–24. https://doi.org/10.4473/TPM.16.1.1

Bracht, E.M., Keng-Highberger, F.T., Avolio, B.J. and Huang Y. (2021) Take a "selfie": Examining how leaders emerge from leader self-awareness, self-leadership, and self-efficacy. *Front. Psychol.* 12, 635085. https://doi.org/0.3389/fpsyg.2021.635085

Bush, S., Michalek, D. and Francis L. (2020) Perceived leadership styles, outcomes of leadership, and self-efficacy among nurse leaders: A hospital-based survey to inform leadership development at a US regional medical center. *Nurse Lead*. 10.1016/j.mnl.2020.07.010. Epub ahead of print. PMID: 33024420; PMCID: PMC7529370.

Datta, B. (2015) Assessing the effectiveness of authentic leadership. *International Journal of Leadership Studies*, 9(1), 62–75.

Day David, V., Fleenor John, W., Atwater Leanne, E., Sturm Rachel, E. and McKee Rob, A., (2014) Advances in leader and leadership development: A review of 25years of research and theory. *The Leadership Quarterly*, 25, 1, 63–82, ISSN 1048–9843, https://doi.org/10.1016/j.leaqua.2013.11.004.

Dubey, P., Pathak, A. K. and Sahu, K. K. (2023) Assessing the influence of effective leadership on job satisfaction and organisational citizenship behaviour, *Rajagiri Management Journal*, 17(3), 221–237. https://doi.org/10.1108/RAMJ-07-2022-0108

Dwyer, L.P. (2019) Leadership self-efficacy: Review and leader development implications. *Journal of Management Development*, 38(8), 637–650. https://doi.org/10.1108/JMD-03-2019-0073

Gabriel, Peace Ifidon, Biriowu Chris Samuel. and Dagogo Eli Legg-Jack. (2020) Examining succession and replacement planning in work organizations. *European Journal of Business Management and Research*. 5(2). http://dx.doi.org/10.24018/ejbmr.2020.5.2.192.

Gardner William, L., Karam Elizabeth, P., Alvesson Mats. and Einola Katja. (2021) Authentic leadership theory: The case for and against, *The Leadership Quarterly*. 32(6), 101495, ISSN 1048–9843. https://doi.org/10.1016/j.leaqua.2021.101495

Gutterman, A. (2023) Leadership Traits and Attributes. SSRN: https://ssrn.com/abstract=4560190

Hargett, C. W., Doty, J. P., Hauck, J. N., Webb, A. M., Cook, S. H., Tsipis, N. E. and Taylor, D. C. (2017) Developing a model for effective leadership in healthcare: A concept mapping approach. *Journal of Healthcare Leadership*, 9, 69–78. https://doi.org/10.2147/JHL.S141664

Hoang, G., Luu, T. T. and Yang, M. (2025) A systematic literature review of authentic leadership in tourism and hospitality: A call for future research. *Cornell Hospitality Quarterly*, 66(1), 110–132. https://doi.org/10.1177/19389655241241471

Hughes, V (2018) What are the barriers to effective nurse leadership? A review. *Athens Journal of Health*, 5(1), 7–20. https://doi.org/10.30958/ajh.5-1-1 doi=10.30958/ajh.5–1–1

Jafarinia, S., Kheirandish, M., Hassanpoor, A. and Bakhshandeh, S. (2019) Identifying work expectations of millennial generation in workplace by using meta-synthesis. *Public Organizations Management*, 7(4), 11–24.

Jujuk Novi, R. R. and Tridayanti Hermien. (2024) The Influenz of Gen X And Gen Y on motivation by leadership style. *International Journal of Entrepreneurship and Business Development*, 7, 4; 848–861. ISSN: 2597–4785

Kane, A., Yarker, J. and Lewis, R. (2021) Measuring self-confidence in workplace settings: A conceptual and methodological review of measures of self-confidence, self-efficacy and self-esteem. *International Coaching Psychology Review*, 16(1), 67–89.

Klug, K., Felfe, J. and Krick, A. (2022) Does self-care make you a better leader? A multisource study linking leader self-care to health-oriented leadership, employee self-care, and health. *International Journal of Environmental Research and Public Health*, 19(11), 6733. https://doi.org/10.3390/ijerph19116733

Krampitz, J., Seubert, C., Furtner, M. and Glaser, J. (2021) Self-leadership: A meta-analytic review of intervention effects on leaders' capacities. *Journal of Leadership Studies*, 15, 21–39. https://doi.org/10.1002/jls.21782

Lartey Sarah, A., Montgomery Carmel, L., Olson Joanne, K. and Cummings Greta, G. (2023) Leadership self-efficacy and nurses' aspiration to leadership: An evolutionary concept analysis. *International Journal of Nursing Studies*, 143, 104496, ISSN 0020–7489. https://doi.org/10.1016/j.ijnurstu.2023.104496.

Lee, C. (1989) Theoretical weaknesses lead to practical problems: the example of self-efficacy theory. *J Behav Ther Exp Psychiatry*. 20(2), 115–23. https://doi.org/10.1016/0005-7916(89)90044-x. PMID: 2685044.

Liou, Y.-H. and Daly, A. J. (2020) Investigating leader self-efficacy through policy engagement and social network position. *Educational Policy*, 34(3), 411–448. https://doi.org/10.1177/0895904818773904

Machida Moe. and Schaubroeck John. (2011) The role of self-efficacy beliefs in leader development. *Journal of Leadership & Organizational Studies*, 18, 459. https://doi.org/10.1177/1548051811404419

Ocho, Oscar Noel, Pieper Barbara, Pulcini Joyce. and Wheeler Erica. (2020a) Nursing leadership in a pandemic: Lessons learned from COVID-19 – An opinion. *World Council of Enterostomal Therapists Journal*. 40(3), 43–46. https://doi.org/10.33235/wcet.40.3.43-46.

Ocho, O. N., Wheeler, E., Sheppard, C., Caesar-Greasley, L. A., Rigby, J. and Tomblin Murphy, G. (2020b). Nurses' preparation for transitioning into positions of leadership-A Caribbean perspective. *J Nurs Manag*. 28(6), 1356–1363. https://doi.org/10.1111/jonm.13089. Epub 2020 Aug 4. PMID: 32671889.

Rahayu, J. N. and Tridayanti, H. (2024). The influenz of gen X And gen Y on motivation by leadership style. *IJEBD (International Journal of Entrepreneurship and Business Development)*. 7(4), 848–861.

Saakvitne, K. W. and Pearlman, L. A. (1996). *Transforming the pain: A workbook on vicarious traumatization for helping professionals who work with traumatized clients*. New York, NY: W. W. Norton & Company, pp. 61–66, 93–95 in Khan Katija (2022 unpublished), Mental Health Toolkit For Health Professionals, University of the West Indies School of Nursing.

Siciliano, M. D. (2016) It's the quality not the quantity of ties that matters: Social networks and self-efficacy beliefs. *American Educational Research Journal*, 53(2), 227–262.

Urick, A., Carpenter B. W. and Eckert, J. (2021) Confronting COVID: Crisis leadership, turbulence, and self-care. *Front. Educ*. 6, 642861. https://doi.org/10.3389/feduc.2021.642861

Chapter 3
Deep level well-being
Compassion and self-compassion

Ann Jackson

INTRODUCTION

The NHS Long Term Workforce Plan (2023a), and the NHS Well-Being Framework (2021), put staff health and well-being as a central part of workforce planning. However, with the change in UK Government in 2024, concern for the difficulties associated with recruitment and retention of key clinical staff, now and in the future, will be paramount, as policy changes indicate a move away from hospital-based care to community-focused health provision. Yet the health and well-being of the workplace should remain a pressing concern for both governments and employing health and care organisations. Therefore, a sustained and targeted approach towards the health and well-being of the workforce is required.

Health and care staff morale is reported to be consistently low and has worsened with the Covid-19 pandemic, which has had a significant and potentially long-lasting impact on staff's ability to continue to go above and beyond. This is having a long-term impact on our health and well-being. Clearly, given the state of the NHS and the unprecedented challenges, strategies for structural service reform need to sit alongside issues relating to staff morale and reported burnout, plus the need to retain, recruit, support and develop the workforce. Particularly in mental health settings, there is a 'wide gap between need and resources' (Darzi, 2024) which makes this a most challenging time. It is imperative to plan effectively to protect the workforce and at the same time ensure a safe and quality care delivery for all of us as citizens and as patients (HEE, 2019).

This chapter explores the potential that compassion and self-compassion strategies offer in the workplace, to support staff at a deep level, in order that they can be truly present and reciprocate compassion in their interactions

DOI: 10.4324/9781041057956-4

and relationships with both patients and colleagues. Whilst the chapter is focused largely on the mental health of health professions, compassion and self-compassion are important for all public sector workers, particularly where there is exposure to the suffering and trauma of others, which is common in all clinical settings, increasingly found in education and significantly in mental health settings. It will explore the benefits of compassion and self-compassion in the context of NHS well-being, the need to preserve the mental health and well-being of the workforce, and at the same time, the need to work harder to prevent burnout and suicide in a post-Covid world. Finally, we will discuss the potential for 'compassionate leadership' to provide the necessary underpinning values and architecture for organisational and system change.

CASE STUDY

As an experienced mental health nurse, although it is many years since I have worked clinically in direct service to patients, clients and service users, my work involves compassion. For over four decades I have worked in various roles as a facilitator of practice development, in policy development and in senior leadership roles, inside and outside of the NHS. I have continually worked with mental health practitioners and have spent many years in provider services.

During Covid-19, I was in a lead role for suicide prevention in a local NHS mental health and community service Trust. Like many other colleagues, on March 23, 2020, when the first national lockdown was announced, there was no real sense of what was to occur, or how this would effect the incidence of local, national and global suicide. There was a lack of any specific evidence or immediate national guidance to predict in any meaningful way what the consequences of a pandemic might have on our understanding of suicide in such a crisis. My colleague, the Police Lead for Suicide Prevention, and I were part of an active local and regional network which meant we were well connected to the developing national discussion. The full story of how we managed to navigate this uncertainty is not documented here, but I have been able to consider in more depth the impact of that experience.

The local public health body, along with myself and the police suicide prevention lead, were able to work collaboratively and met regularly with system partners to implement the practical local strategies we created, built on good intelligence. We were also able to pay attention to articulate and describe our individual and shared experiences, expressing the emotional weight of this time.

First, we were fearful for people already living in poor mental health who were, and those who were not, in contact with mental health services and for those who might be hit hard by the unknown consequences of Covid-19. We knew from previous research that there were established risk factors associated with previous infectious pandemics and that we were applying general population data to local and individual incidences of death by suicide.

Second, we focused on the routine collection of data associated with suicide prevention, and developed new sources of information where none existed, so that we could identify early any local and emerging themes. We became increasingly vigilant and immediately responsive to presenting information relating to deaths by suspected suicide as they came through in the form of incident notifications. We would share this information between the two of us, and I would instigate informing Trust directors and a new process of rapid clinical review. These incident notifications and the necessary actions were received across all hours of the day and night in quite small weekly numbers, but we largely failed to set any parameters around our working hours. There were not as many as we feared, as the numbers of deaths actually remained relatively stable; but we often wondered how we would endure our feelings of overwhelming responsibility in such uncharted territory.

Third, whilst we worked (safely) at home, we were in awe of the front-line, clinical and public service staff who were directly managing complex health delivery, developing responsive services and risking their own health to be with those patients requiring face-to-face care. Who were we to worry about ourselves when colleagues were doing the 'really hard work'? As the early days of the national lockdown turned into weeks and months, our working and non-working lives began to look and feel like a new 'normal'.

We later claimed this period as 'intense'. There was a lack of formal support (especially for those working at home), and we often cited the validation of each other and our collective effort as essential for our own sense of survival, well-being and recovery. Compassion in action.

CRITICAL QUESTIONS

1. What workplace-related and personal stressors can you observe in this case study?
2. What kind of workplace support might have been helpful and in what way?
3. What healthy strategies might have been adopted?
4. What vulnerabilities and emotional challenges are evident in the case study?
5. Where and how might self-compassion be useful in this situation?

COVID-19'S IMPACT ON HEALTH AND WELL-BEING, BURNOUT AND RESILIENCE

It is well documented that pre-Covid, health and care workers were already experiencing high stress levels, staffing shortages, high sickness rates and long-term sickness due to mental health issues (NHS Digital, 2023), plus high workloads, reports of care not given and high rates of reported bullying and harassment occurring in the workplace. Research undertaken during the Covid-19 pandemic was consistent in identifying increased workload, uncertainty, redeployment, stressful and high-risk work environments, with a significant number of health and care workers both in the UK and across the world reporting increased signs of burnout, emotional exhaustion, symptoms of depression, anxiety and post-traumatic stress disorder (PTSD) (WISH, 2022).

Greenberg et al, (2020) described how ethical dilemmas that arose under crisis standards amounted to an 'emotional toll' with long-term moral distress. Coimbra et al, (2024) reported moral distress/injury and suicidality was associated with increased experiences of stress and poor mental health. Several authors reported on the challenges associated with supporting health and well-being staff during these turbulent times, identifying need for informal and formal support mechanisms, but difficulties in accessing this support (Maben et al, 2022) plus the need for emotional support to enhance personal and collective resilience (de Zulueta, 2021). Concern has been raised relating to a Covid-19 'aftermath' and the need for investment to promote a culture that is both compassionate and addresses the systemic issues related to inadequate staffing and high workloads

(Kinman et al, 2020b); they also raised the difficult issue of increased trauma and suicidality during this time and beyond. Likewise, Aloweni et al, (2022) have called for planning that takes account of the prolonged nature of burnout.

However, it is important to recognise the dangers inherent in discussions relating to prevention of burnout and strategies to build resilience. Many authors have sought to ensure that we do not limit our understanding to deficits of failures at the individual level and that root causes and conditions that cause stressors need to be addressed (WISH, 2022; Kinman et al, 2023). Grant and Kinman (2013) reminded us many years ago that 'even highly emotionally resilient professionals' need fully resourced support to undergo their role function adequately.

The next section will explore the extent to which compassion and self-compassion in practice and in the workplace can offer us as an antidote to what de Zulueta (2016) has called 'anxiety-laden contexts'.

COMPASSION AND SELF-COMPASSION IN PRACTICE AND IN THE WORKPLACE

For the purposes of this discussion, we are using the following definition of compassion as described by Paul Gilbert as: "A sensitivity to suffering in **self** and **others** with a **commitment** to try to **alleviate** and **prevent** it" (quotation via the Compassionate Mind Foundation website www.compassionatemind.co.uk).

Professor Paul Gilbert is credited a major contributor to the robust theory base for compassion in healthcare practice in the UK. Importantly, neuroscience has provided evidence on how disruption in the brain's emotional regulation systems has led us to hyperfocus on threat whilst disregarding the need to self-soothe (c.f., Ashar et al., 2016; Davidson and Begley, 2012). This is a simple description offered here, suffice it to say, that whilst we have a lot more evidence on the benefits of compassion on the body, brain and emotions, it is highly complex and continues to receive challenges around

- conceptual clarity and evidence-based interventions to promote compassionate care (Blomberg et al, 2016);
- developing a language to describe compassionate care (Crawford et al, 2013),
- measuring compassionate care (Gilbert et al, 2017); and
- training, supporting and operationalising compassionate care (Egan et al, 2017).

In developing compassionate competency, Gilbert et al, (2017) describes the complexity of developing measures of the 'three orientations and directional flows':

1. The compassion we feel for other people
2. Our experience of compassion from other people
3. Self-compassion

Egan et al, (2018) highlighted that healthcare professionals and students in their study on delivery of compassionate care were not tired of being compassionate but of overcoming the barriers to remaining compassionate. In their study, four themes were identified as

1. keeping it real, the need for authentic compassion;
2. compassion takes time: barriers to delivering compassionate care;
3. no time to think about myself: self-compassion, self-care and health behaviours; and
4. does anybody care?

Sinclair et al, (2016) described the importance of reflective learning and self-awareness as teaching methods, noting that compassion is highly individualised to students and their patients. This need for individual consideration is highlighted further if we consider the need to understand the impact and health consequences of inequality. Sengupta and Saxena (2024) remind us of that 'ethnocultural' differences influence the levels of compassion competency and how a society perceives and interprets suffering determines the course of compassionate action. However, in spite of the challenges, there is now a body of literature and evidence about the benefits of compassionate training, support and reflection for both healthcare professionals and patients.

In mental health settings particularly, healthcare workers are exposed to high levels of distress, people with trauma histories (including staff) who may display behaviours that can be difficult to respond to with compassion. This is the challenge, developing compassionate ways where emotions of staff (Gilbert, 2009; de Zulueta, 2016) and people receiving care can potentially be overwhelming and where the resources for support and supervision are limited.

Gilbert (2009) offers the following:

> *so we can see that compassionate behaviour can be more difficult than it at first appears. It can be tough on us because there are all sorts of dilemmas*

that we have to face; it can be tough on us because it calls on our courage; it can be tough on us because we have to face our own powerful internal emotions; it can be tough on us because it's not always clear what the compassionate way actually is. So the only thing we can do is to be compassionate to the fact that behaving compassionately and facing up to our powerful emotions is tough on us and we can only do our best.

(Gilbert, 2009:pp 443)

West et al. (2020), in an important review of the consequences of poor mental health and well-being in doctors, nurses and midwives, developed the following ABC framework of core work needs – with the three need areas of (1) autonomy, (2) belonging and (3) connection and the eight recommendations:

Worline and Dutton (2017), in their work 'awakening compassion at work', suggest that we need to develop more generous interpretations of 'suffering'; that there are three forms of this – withholding blame, imbuing with worth and cultivating presence. In believing that a) everyone is worthy of compassion, and b) that someone's presentation of suffering is real, it is often difficult to be generous when

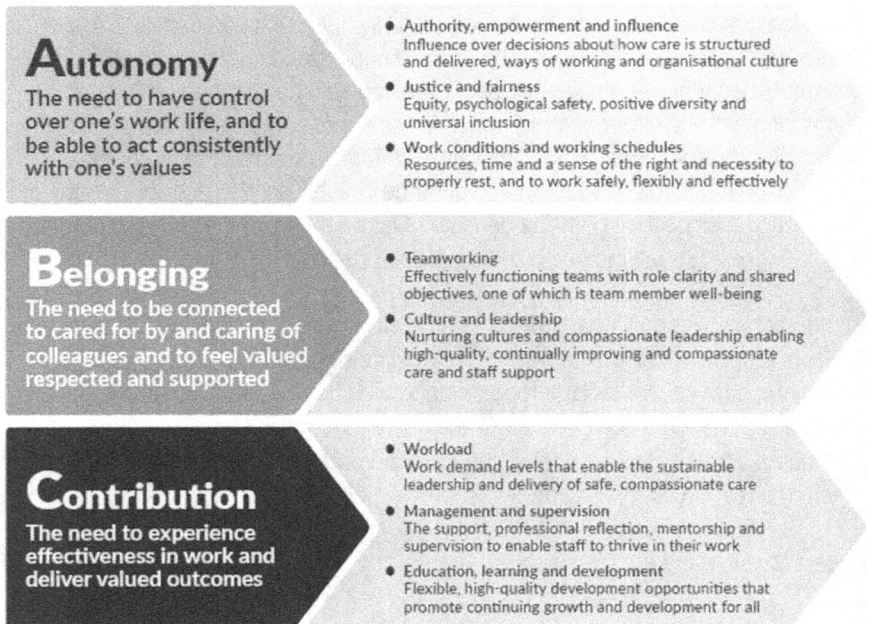

Autonomy
The need to have control over one's work life, and to be able to act consistently with one's values

- Authority, empowerment and influence
  Influence over decisions about how care is structured and delivered, ways of working and organisational culture
- Justice and fairness
  Equity, psychological safety, positive diversity and universal inclusion
- Work conditions and working schedules
  Resources, time and a sense of the right and necessity to properly rest, and to work safely, flexibly and effectively

Belonging
The need to be connected to cared for by and caring of colleagues and to feel valued respected and supported

- Teamworking
  Effectively functioning teams with role clarity and shared objectives, one of which is team member well-being
- Culture and leadership
  Nurturing cultures and compassionate leadership enabling high-quality, continually improving and compassionate care and staff support

Contribution
The need to experience effectiveness in work and deliver valued outcomes

- Workload
  Work demand levels that enable the sustainable leadership and delivery of safe, compassionate care
- Management and supervision
  The support, professional reflection, mentorship and supervision to enable staff to thrive in their work
- Education, learning and development
  Flexible, high-quality development opportunities that promote continuing growth and development for all

Figure 3.1 The ABC of core work needs (West, M., Bailey, S., and Williams, E. (2020). The courage of compassion: Supporting Nurses and Midwives to Deliver High-Quality Care. London: The King's Fund, London.)

there is poor performance, incivility and bullying. Accountability is important here, as acting with compassion is not about merely a personal quality of 'niceness' and 'being kind'; it is also vigorously about maintaining high standards and holding people to account. The importance of being able to engage in difficult conversations, saying the hard things and at the same time withholding blame and judgement demonstrates both skills and courage.

Reflective task [1]

Think about the four attributes of compassion in an organisation, as outlined by West (2021):

1. **Attending:** noticing suffering, difficulties and challenges at work (your own and others')
2. **Understanding:** being curious, withholding blame, focusing on 'What's the learning here?'
3. **Empathising:** being aware of continually changing conditions in yourself and others, developing empathic listening and tuning in to feelings of concern
4. **Helping:** directing your efforts towards what is most helpful in alleviating others' suffering

Then consider the following:

- How well do you notice aspects of behaviours that might alert you that someone is suffering?
- How good are you at noticing your own difficulties?
- How comfortable are you in hearing about colleagues' vulnerabilities and suffering?
- Do you take time to listen to yourself and others?
- How prepared and confident are you that you can respond to understand with empathy and without judgement?
- Do you always take the opportunity to act on the needs of others?
- Do you act on your own needs?

THE IMPORTANCE OF SELF-COMPASSION: TENDER AND FIERCE, AND PREVENTION OF BURNOUT

Michael West (2021), amongst others, has claimed that compassion is an antidote to burnout. Given that we are concerned with the health and well-being of healthcare professionals, particularly in the prevention of burnout and empathy or compassion fatigue, what sources of support can we develop for ourselves?

Kristin Neff developed the self-compassion scale in 2003 and can be freely accessed in the link provided in the Learning Resources section. Her work is important in understanding how, as a core element of compassion, self-compassion is a necessary level of awareness (of self and of the reality of our situations) and acceptance (that we are only human). She suggests that "when we see our situation with clarity and objectivity, we open the door to wisdom". Neff (2011; p 41) outlines three broad aspects of self-compassion:

1. Self-kindness – that we be gentle and understanding with ourselves, rather than harshly critical and judgemental
2. Common humanity – feeling connected with others in the experience of life rather than feeling isolated and alienated by our suffering
3. Mindfulness – that we hold our experience in balanced awareness, rather than ignoring our pain or exaggerating it

If we take self kindness, particularly as this might be more difficult for professional to develop. They are perhaps conditioned by expectation of being the giver of compassion and not always so good at taking care of themselves. Neff says:

> *Self-kindness, by definition, means that we stop the constant self-judgement and disparaging internal commentary that most of us have come to see as normal, it requires us to understand our foibles and failures instead of condemning them and self-kindness involves more than merely stopping self-judgment. It involves actively comforting ourselves.*
>
> (Neff, 2011:p 14)

Self-compassion then means talking to and treating ourselves as we would a friend. Neff (2021) distinguishes between tender and fierce self-compassion, both of which are helpful for healthcare settings. She suggests that these should be in balance; tender self-compassion described as soothing and calming actions as described earlier, and 'fierce', where there are actions to draw boundaries, protect self from harm, stand up for oneself and fight for resources. Where healthcare professionals see themselves as activists for social justice and equality, it is even more important to understand the emotional impact and do work to foster strength in the face of structural inequalities and barriers. Fierce self-compassion therefore "allows us to see our problems clearly, feel empowered by our sense of connection to others and find the courage to act" (Neff and Germer, 2024). This is important in the prevention of burnout, secondary traumatic stress and empathy fatigue. An important aspect is the need for healthcare professionals to sometimes take too much responsibility for things beyond their control.

Neff and Germer (2024) offer an insightful thought:

> *The wisdom of self-compassion reminds us that we have human limitations, and although we can try our best, we don't have power over the mental, psychological or physical health of others. Self-compassion allows us to be humble and give up the illusion of control.*
>
> (Neff and Germer, 2024; p99)

Egan et al. (2017), amongst others, argue for self-compassion training to run alongside that of compassion. They have also suggested that given the evidence of the benefit of mindfulness, self-compassion and self-care, it is harmful *not* to implement them into the healthcare workplace. Kinman (2022) suggest a personal self-care toolbox as part of an overall approach to developing strategies for well-being. Miley et al. (2024) have reported that self-compassion had a positive influence on the relationship between perceived clinical decision-making ability and moral distress.

Reflective task [2]

Consider the three elements of self-compassion as offered by Neff (2003, 2011):

1. Mindfulness
2. Common humanity
3. Self-kindness

Reflect on the following questions:

1. To what extent do you regularly ask yourself, 'What do I need right now?'?
2. Do you notice your inner critic/negative or harsh self-talk?
3. How mindful or aware are you of the reality of your situation in your personal life or in the workplace?
4. Are you able to offer yourself the same kindness that you would give to a friend in need?
5. How can you be gentle with yourself as you work through your difficulties and challenges?
6. If you could let go of the pressures to be perfect, what would feel like a kind first step?
7. How do you create safe spaces for yourself and others?
8. Are we doing enough to support staff when they are already burned out, mentally unwell and distressed?

The next section with look briefly at the very difficult area of suicide prevention in the healthcare workplace.

COMPASSIONATE WORKPLACES AND SUICIDE PREVENTION

In response to more recent data from the ONS (2021), some healthcare professionals are considered to be at 24% higher risk of suicide than the general population. However, this is mainly because suicides in female nurses are 23% above the national average. NCISH (2020) raised that little is known about the factors that increase the risk to female nurses. However, stressful workplace issues were cited in individual deaths, and there are now two main areas of research. NCISH has been commissioned to conduct a general study of suicides amongst healthcare staff, and there is a specific project to study female nurse suicidality (please see further reading section later). Riley et al. (2023) identified the gendered nature of this urgent research, and Jackson and Worner (in print) have raised an important link between domestic abuse and suicidality.

Riley et al. (2023) state:

> *Framing nurse suicide within the contexts of social, environmental and economic challenges or historical injustices will help us understand the distress, inequality and injustice experienced by the female majority and ethnically diverse nursing workforce.*
>
> (Riley et al, 2023: 1246)

Two further resources have been developed:

1.   NHS (2023c) National Suicide Prevention Toolkit for England
2.   NHS employee suicide: a postvention toolkit to help manage the impact and provide support – which offers specific support following the death of a colleague

Both tools are crucial for implementation to ensure that there is a set of guidelines and policy to create a workplace culture that promotes mental well-being, encourages early intervention and supports recovery following traumatic events.

Both compassion for others and self-compassion are vital components in achieving workplaces that are psychologically safe, where there is openness, and individuals can seek help when they are struggling with work-related stress. The suicide prevention toolkit describes the range of workplace resources to consider including access to clinical supervision; extending access to psychological support; management of work-related stress; provision of additional support to those absent from work due to sickness; taking action to prevent bullying; and ensuring additional support is available during times of high additional stress, such as workplace changes, investigating allegations or following serious incidents. In mental health settings, there should be particular concern and follow-up support following the death by suicide of a patient.

Whilst these resources are relatively new, it is important that they become familiar across all settings in order that we can protect staff. It is encouraging that the NHS has mandated the appointment of a board level director known as the Health and Well-being Guardian to oversee principle 2: Will ensure that where there is an individual or team exposure to a clinical event that is particularly distressing, time is made available to check the well-being impact on those NHS staff and learners; and principle 5: The death by suicide of any member of staff or a learner working in an NHS organisation will be independently examined and the findings reported through the Well-being Guardian to the Board.

What kind of support and leadership is required to ensure that the workforce has good health and well-being? The next section will explore compassionate leadership as a solution to some of the difficulties associated with poor health and well-being.

COMPASSIONATE LEADERSHIP – BUILDING THE ARCHITECTURE

In recent years, compassionate and collective leadership in healthcare have become more popular and provided an architecture to support leadership that demonstrates the values and behaviours of compassion. West (2021) has described the four elements of working compassionately as attending, understanding, empathising and helping. Additionally, there are five fundamental factors for a workplace culture that is innovative and provides high-quality care:

- Inspiring vision and strategy
- Clear agreed and aligned goals at every level
- Positive inclusion and participation
- Enthusiastic team and cross-boundary working
- Support and autonomy for staff to innovate

Effective leadership is demonstrated by ensuring clear direction, alignment of objectives that are coordinated and that commitment is nurtured through trust and meeting the ABC (seen earlier in previous section on compassion in the workplace) of core needs.

Worline and Dutton (2017) distinguish between leading *with* and leading *for* compassion. This is summarised as the following:

> *Leaders are the high-level architects of compassion in their organisations. They move people by modelling personal presence in the face of suffering. They foster compassion throughout the system by their capacity to attune to others, feel concern, listen and act with care. Leading with compassion takes on even more power when it is combined with a system-level view of leading for compassion. Leaders who invest in compassion competence and communicate to reinforce shared humanity unlock resources to alleviate suffering.*
>
> (Worline and Dutton, 2017; p 187)

De Zulueta (2016) raises the potential for coaching to be tailored to support the development of compassionate leadership across organisations. She goes on to say:

> *Senior leaders will require the capacity to establish a collective vision to support the greater good, make connections and work across boundaries, tolerate uncertainty, collate multiple perspectives and ensure that leadership is distributed. They will need to embody and model compassionate attitudes and behaviours and receive the support and training to develop and maintain self-compassion and emotional resilience.*
>
> (De Zulueta, 2016; p 7)

De Zulueta (2021) highlighted, particularly during and following the Covid-19 pandemic, for leaders to be highly self-aware, attuned to others, manage their emotions and respond with wisdom in times of crisis.

In addition to the personal qualities and behaviours associated with compassionate leadership, it is imperative to establish systemic needs to develop supportive environments and adequate training (Crawford et al, 2013; Kinman et al, 2020a; Rizal et al, 2021; Howick et al, 2024). Kinman et al., 2020a state: 'fix the workplace, not the worker!'

Finally, it is hard to argue with the following from Michael West (2021):

> *It is the responsibility of all of us to practice compassion, self-compassion and compassionate leadership in our health and social care more widely.*

Our imperative for our future and that of our children and our planet is to lead compassionately to sustain wisdom, humanity and presence for all our futures.

(West, 2021: p 221)

IN SUMMARY

This chapter has focused on a major concern in current health workplaces – the mental, emotional and psychological health of its healthcare professionals. It has sought, at an introductory level, to show a trajectory from before Covid-19 towards a suffering workforce. Workplace conditions were made worse by the experiences of many groups of staff, and we are in a continuing crisis in relation to staffing shortages, high workloads, low morale and burnout. This chapter has outlined a few ideas related to the role of compassion, self-compassion and compassionate leadership in the reduction of burnout and ultimately workplace suicide prevention. Whilst we are now in a post-Covid context, we can anticipate that there will be future pandemics, and it is vitally important that we learn the lessons and have compassionate strategies in place to fully support mental health and well-being in the workplace. It is incumbent on all professional, clinical and managerial staff to take some personal responsibility for their own health and well-being and at the same time become increasingly active as part of the collective leadership of the NHS and other healthcare settings. As we accept our shared and common humanity, inherently flawed, we must endeavour try to connect authentically with people who are suffering, as are we. We are expected to do this in an imperfect system, society and world where vulnerability is yet to be seen as a strength, where inequalities persist and where national policy is uncertain. To make systemic change is to be part of a social movement of compassion, to participate in actions that can work towards the prevention of suffering and injustice.

Therefore, the health and care workforce, educators and leaders need to have the curiosity to notice and name suffering around them. We need to have the complex skills and personal qualities to respond with compassion and to have the courage to always act with integrity and wisdom. To work compassionately is a skill and a choice; it is also a political act.

ADDITIONAL RESOURCES

- Creating a Compassionate World: www.compassionatemind.co.uk
- Dr Kristin Neff: The Self Compassion Test: https://self-compassion.org/self-compassion-test/
- Health and Safety Executive Stress Talking Toolkits: www.hse.gov.uk/stress/talking-toolkit.htm

- NHS England Talking Toolkit: Preventing work -related stress for NHS service providers in England: www.hse.gov.uk/stress/assets/docs/talking-toolkit-nhs-england.pdf
- NHS England The L.O.T.U.S Compassionate Leadership Framework and Toolkit: www.england.nhs.uk/north-west/wp-content/uploads/sites/48/2024/07/11125-ML-NHS-compassionate-toolkit_FINAL-09.07.24.pdf
- The King's Fund; An introduction to leading with kindness and compassion in health and social care: www.kingsfund.org.uk/leadership-development/courses/leading-kindness-compassion-health-social-care
- Revisioning Nurse Distress and Suicidality in women nurses: www.nursesuicidestudy.com

FURTHER READING

Bivins R., Tierney, S. and Seers, K. (2017) Compassionate care: Not easy, not free, not only nurses. *BMJ Qual Saf* 26:1023–1026. https://doi.org/10.1136/bmjqs -2017–007005

BMA. (2021) *Moral Distress and Moral Injury: Recognising and Tackling It for UK Doctors*. London: British Medical Association. Accessible via www.bma.org.uk/media/4209/bma-moral-distress-injury-survey-report-june-2021.pdf (last accessed 10/3/2025)

Crawford P., Brown B., Kvangarsnes M. and Gilbert P. (2014) The design of compassionate care. *Journal of Clinical Nursing* 23(23–24): 3589–3599. https://doi.org/10.1111/jocn.12632

Dahl C., Wilson-Mendenhalla C. and Davidson R. (2020) The plasticity of well-being: A training-based framework for the cultivation of human flourishing. *Perspectives in Biological Sciences*. Posner, M.I., Wilson-Mendhall, C.D. and Davidson R.J (editors). www.pnas.org/cgi/doi/10.1073/pnas.2014859117

HM Government. (2023) Suicide prevention strategy for England: 2023 to 2028 – GOV.UK. www.gov.uk/government/publications/suicide-prevention-strategy-for-england-2023-to-2028 (last accessed 13.01.2025).

Irons, C. and Beaumont, E. (2017) *The Compassionate Mind Workbook, A Step-by-Step Guide to Developing Your Compassionate Self*, Robinson, Great Britain

Kinman, G. and Greenberg, N. (2024) Suicide postvention in the workplace supporting organisations and employees, society of occupational medicine. Accessible via www.som.org.uk/sites/som.org.uk/files/Suicide_Postvention_in_the_Workpace_Supporting_Organisations_and_Employees_2024_09_11.pdf

NHS Digital. (2020) NHS sickness absence rates –Medrxi report – The mental health of staff working in intensive care during COVID-19 Report. Accessible via www.medrxiv.org/content/10.1101/2020.11.03.20208322v2.full.pdf (last accessed 10.3.2025)

NHS England. (2023b) Health and wellbeing guardian guidance: Appendix 1 – early evaluation and recommendations to improve impact and reach. A report published. 11 October, 2023. Accessible via www.england.nhs.uk/long-read/health-and-wellbeing-guardian-guidance-appendix-1-early-evaluation-and-recommendations-to-improve-impact-and-reach/ (last accessed 10.3.2025)

NHS England. (2023c) Working together to prevent suicide in the NHS workforce. A toolkit. Accessible via www.england.nhs.uk/publication/working-together-to-prevent-suicide-in-the-nhs/ (last accessed 10.3.2025).

Revisioning Distress and Suicidality in Women Nurses. (2024) A nurse suicide sudy suffering with suicide: Revisioning distress and suicidality in women nurses. Accessible via www.nursesuicidestudy.com/project (last accessed 13.01.2025)

Traynor, M. (2023). Empathy, caring and compassion: Toward a Freudian critique of nursing work. *Nursing Philosophy*, 24: e12399. https://doi.org/10.1111/nup.12399

World Health Organization. (2021) Comprehensive mental health action plan 2013–2030. Geneva: World Health Organization. Accessible via www.who.int/publications/i/item/9789240031029 (last accessed 10.3.2025)

REFERENCES

Aloweni F., Ayre T., Teo I., Tan H. and Lim S.H. (2022) A year after COVID-19: Its impact on nurses' psychological well-being. *Journal of Nursing Management*, 1–12. https://doi.org/10.1111/jonm.13814

Ashar, Y.K., Andrews-Hanna, J.R., Dimidjian, S. and Wager, T.D. (2016) *Toward a Neuroscience of Compassion: A brain systems-based model and research agenda*. Chapter 8 in Positive Neuroscience. Greene, J.D., Morrison, I. and Seligman, M.E.P (Editors). Oxford University Press. https://doi.org/10.1093/acprof:oso/9780199977925.003.0009

Blomberg K., Griffiths P., Wengstrom Y., May, C. and Bridges, J. (2016) Interventions for compassionate nursing care: A systematic review. *International Journal of Nursing Studies* 62: 137–155

Coimbra B.M., Zylberstajn C., van Zuiden M., Hoeboer C.M., Mello A.F., Mello M.F. and Olff M. (2024) Moral injury and mental health among health-care workers during the COVID-19 pandemic: Meta-analysis. *Eur J Psychotraumatol*. 15(1):2299659. https://doi.org/10.1080/20008066.2023.2299659. Epub 2024 Jan 8. PMID: 38189775; PMCID: PMC10776063. https://pmc.ncbi.nlm.nih.gov/articles/PMC10776063/pdf/ZEPT_15_2299659.pdf

Crawford P., Gilbert P., Gilbert J., Gale C. and Harvey K. (2013) The language of compassion in acute mental health care. *Qualitative Health Research* 23(6):719–727. https://citeseerx.ist.psu.edu/document?repid=rep1&type=pdf&doi=37520247e8bfb6b04520ccce56d8758033c1d13d

Darzi A. (2024) Independent investigation of the National Health Service. September 2024 Open Government License. Accessible via https://assets.publishing.service.gov.uk/media/66f42ae630536cb92748271f/Lord-Darzi-Independent-Investigation-of-the-National-Health-Service-in-England-Updated-25-September.pdf (last accessed 19/2/2025).

Davidson R. and Begley S. (2012) *The Emotional Life of Your Brain*, Hudson Street Press, New York: NY.

de Zulueta P. (2016) Developing compassionate leadership in health care: An integrative review. *Journal of Healthcare Leadership* (8):1–10 https://doi.org/10.2147/JHL.S93724

de Zulueta P. (2021) How do we sustain compassionate healthcare? Compassionate leadership in the time of the COVID-19 pandemic. *Clinics in Integrated Care* 8. https://doi.org/10.1016/j.intcar.2021.100071

Egan H., Mantzios M. and Jackson C. (2017) Health Practitioners and the directive towards compassionate healthcare in the UK: exploring the need to educate health practitioners on how to be self-compassionate and mindful alongside mandating compassion towards patients. *Health Professions Education* 3:61–63. https://doi.org/10.1016/j.hpe.2016.09.002

Egan, H., Keyte, R., McGowan, K., Peters, L., Lemon, N., Parsons, S., Meadows, S., Fardy, T., Singh, P. and Mantzios, M., (2019) 'You before me': A qualitative study of health care professionals' and students' understanding and experiences of compassion in the workplace, self-compassion, self-care and health behaviours. *Health Professions Education*, 5(3): 225–236.

Gilbert P. (2009) *The Compassionate Mind*, Robinson, Great Britain.

Gilbert P., Catarino F., Duarte C., Matos M., Kolt R., Stubbs J., Ceresatto L., Duarte J., Pinto-Gouveia J. and Basran J. (2017) The development of compassionate engagement and action scales for self and others. *Journal of Compassionate Health Care* 4:4. https://doi.org/10.1186/s40639-017-0033-3

Grant, L. and Kinman, G (2013) *The importance of emotional resilience for staff and students in the 'helping' professions: developing an emotional curriculum*. The Higher Education Academy – research briefing. Accessible via www.advance-he.ac.uk/knowledge-hub/importance-emotional-resilience-staff-and-students-helping-professions-developing (last accessed 10.3.2025)

Greenberg N., Docherty M., Gnanapragasam S. and Wessely, S. (2020) Managing mental health challenges faced by healthcare workers during covid-19 pandemic. *BMJ*. https://doi.org/10.1136/bmj.m1211

Health Education England. (2019) NHS staff and learners' mental well-being Commission. February 2019. Accessible via www.hee.nhs.uk/sites/default/files/documents/NHS%20%28HEE%29%20-%20Mental%20Wellbeing%20Commission%20Report.pdf (last accessed 10.3.2025)

Howick J., de Zulueta P. and Muir G. (2024) Beyond empathy training for practitioners: Cultivating empathic healthcare systems and leadership. *Journal of Evaluation in Clinical Practice* 30(4):548–558. https://doi.org/10.1111/jep.13970

Irons, C. and Beaumont, E. (2017) *The Compassionate Mind Workbook*, Robinson, Great Britian. ISBN 978-1-4721-3590-2

Kinman G. (2022) Research in practice – supporting practitioner well-being. Accessible via www.researchinpractice.org.uk/

Kinman Gail, Dovey Ian. and Teoh Kevin. (2023) Burnout in healthcare, risks and solutions, The society of occupational medicine. Accessible via www.som.org.uk/sites/som.org.uk/files/Burnout_in_healthcare_risk_factors_and_solutions_July2023_0.pdf (last accessed 10.3.2025)

Kinman G., Teoh, K. and Harriss A. (2020a) Improving the mental health and well-being of nurses and midwives. July 2020. Report accessible via www.som.org.uk/sites/som.org.uk/files/The_Mental_Health_and_Wellbeing_of_Nurses_and_Midwives_in_the_United_Kingdom.pdf (last accessed 10.3.2025)

Kinman G., Teoh K. and Harriss A. (2020b) Supporting the well-being of healthcare workers during and after COVID-19, (editorial). *Occupational Medicine*. https://doi.org/10.1093/occmed/kqaa096

Maben J., Conolly A., Abrams R., Rowland E., Harris R., Kelly D., Kent B. and Couper K. (2022) 'You can't walk through water without getting wet' UK nurses' distress and psychological health needs during the Covid-19 pandemic: A longitudinal interview study. *International Journal of International Studies* 131:104242. https://doi.org/10.1016/j.ijnurstu.2022.104242

Miley M., Mantzios M., Egan H. and Connabeer K. (2024) Exploring the moderating role of health-promoting behaviours and self-compassion on the relationship between clinical decision-making and nurses' well-being. *Journal of Research in Nursing* 1–13. https://doi.org/10.1177/17449871241270822

NCISH. (2020) Suicide by female nurses: An brief report. University of Manchester. Accessible via https://documents.manchester.ac.uk/display.aspx?DocID=49577 (last accessed 10.3.2025)

Neff, K. (2003) Self-compassion: An alternative conceptualization of a healthy attitude toward oneself. *Self and identity* 2(2): 85–101.

Neff, K. (2011) *Self-Compassion, Stop Beating Yourself up and Leave Security Behind*, Wiliam Morris, Great Britian.

Neff K. (2021) *Fierce Self-Compassion – How Women can Harness Kindness to Speak up, Claim their Power and Thrive*, Penguin Life, Great Britian.

Neff, K. and Germer, Christopher. (2024) *Mindful Self-Compassion for Burnout*. The Guildford Press, New York, NY

NHS. (2020) The NHS people plan we are the NHS: People plan for 2020/2021 – action for us all. A report July 2020. Accessible via www.england.nhs.uk/wp-content/uploads/2020/07/We-Are-The-NHS-Action-For-All-Of-Us-FINAL-March-21.pdf (last accessed 10.3.2025)

NHS Digital. (2023) 'NHS sickness absence rates, August 2022'. 30 April 2009 to 31 August 2022. Accessible via https://digital.nhs.uk/data-and-information/publications/statistical/nhs

NHS England. (2023a) NHS long term workforce plan June 20230. Accessible via www.england.nhs.uk/wp-content/uploads/2023/06/nhs-long-term-workforce-plan-v1.21.pdf

NHS (2023c) National Suicide Prevention Toolkit for England. Available via https://www.england.nhs.uk/publication/working-together-to-prevent-suicide-in-the-nhs/ (last accessed 6/10/2025)

NHS Health and Well-being Strategic Overview. (2021) Creating a health and well-being culture. A resource tool kit. Accessible via www.england.nhs.uk/wp-content/uploads/2021/11/NHS-health-and-wellbeing-framework-strategic-overview.pdf (last accessed 10.3.2025)

ONS. (2021) Suicide by occupation, England: 2011 to 2015. Accessible via www.ons.gov.uk/peoplepopulationandcommunity/birthsdeathsandmarriages/deaths/articles/suicidebyoccupation/england2011to2015 (last accessed 10.3.2025)

Riley R., Causer H., Patrick L. and Rogowsky R. (2023) Why are dominant suicidology approaches failing nurses? A call for a feminist critical suicidology perspective (Editorial). *Journal of Advanced Nursing*. https://doi.org/10.1111/jan.15899

Rizal F., Egan H. and Mantzios M. (2021) Mindfulness, compassion, and self-compassion as moderator of environmental support on competency in mental health nursing. SN *Comprehensive Clinical Medicine* 3:1534–1543. https://doi.org/10.1007/s42399-021-00904-5

Sengupta P. and Saxena P. (2024) The art of compassion in mental healthcare for all: Back to the basics. *Indian J Psychol Med*. 46(1):72–77

Sinclair S., Norris J., McConnell S., Harvey M., Chochinov H., Hack T., Hagen N., McClement S. and Bouchal S. (2016) Compassion: A scoping review of the healthcare literature.

BMC Palliative Care 15:6. https://doi.org/10.1186/s12904-016-0080-0 (last accessed 23.01.2023)

West M., Bailey, S. and Williams, E. (2020) *The Courage of Compassion (2020) Supporting Nurses and Midwives to Deliver High-Quality Care*. London: The Kings Fund. Accessible via www.kingsfund.org.uk/insight-and-analysis/reports/courage-compassion-supporting-nurses-midwives (last accessed 10.3.2025)

West M. (2021) *Compassionate Leadership – Sustaining Wisdom, Humanity and Presence in Health and Social Care*, Swirling Leaf Press. ISBN 0995766975

WISH. (2022) Forum on the mental health of health and care workers our duty of care a global call to action to protect the mental health of health and care workers. Accessible via https://cdn.who.int/media/docs/default-source/health-workforce/working4health/20221005-wish-duty.pdf?sfvrsn=a021c187_7&download=true (last accessed 10.3.2025)

Worline M. and Dutton J. (2017) *Awakening Compassion at Work*, Berrett-Koehler publishers, Canada

Chapter 4

Lessons for leading well and living well

A personal reflection

Alice Webster

INTRODUCTION

In today's fast-paced world, the concepts of leading well and living well are increasingly intertwined. Balancing professional responsibilities with personal life is a significant challenge for leaders of any level. Friedman (2008) suggests that leaders who achieve work-life balance are more effective and sustainable in their roles. These are individuals who avoid burnout and maintain their well-being, positively influencing their own and others' own leadership capabilities. Effective leadership extends beyond professional success, encompassing personal growth and well-being.

This chapter is a personal reflection that explores how leading with integrity, empathy, and balance can enhance both personal and professional lives. It draws upon my own experiences, of good and bad leadership, and that leadership is not merely unidimensional when viewing the vast amounts of leadership literature evidence available. Strong and effective leadership is about collaboration, not control. This chapter, therefore, is based upon personal reflections on leading well and living well, exploring the interconnectedness of effective leadership and a fulfilling professional life.

THE QUALITIES OF EFFECTIVE LEADERSHIP

The wind blew gently
taking away all that needed to be changed.
The tide washed at my feet,
sand trickled through my toes, and I sank a little deeper.

DOI: 10.4324/9781041057956-5

Taking a deep breath,
I realized that everything I needed
to nurture and develop is within me.
I felt the fragility of this moment deep inside,
along with the anticipation
waiting to be released.

Realising and releasing inner strength (as outlined in the poem I wrote earlier) is something that many of us hold onto and often succeed in channelling, just when one least expects to. Leading well requires a foundation of integrity and authenticity. According to Covey (2004), effective leaders prioritise principles over tactics, ensuring their actions align with their core values. This alignment fosters trust and respect among team members, which is essential for successful leadership.

In the fast-paced world we operate in, the way in which we both lead and are led can have extreme responses, can also form that which sees one thrive, to a very negative personal impact when one's own values are so significantly challenged that the inner core of what makes you 'you' is adversely affected. Working in situations where this occurs is not uncommon and will undoubtedly happen at some point in your professional life.

REFLECTION

- Harmony is not something that is achievable 100 percent of the time. How do you manage this?
- Where and how do you seek harmonious living, in getting the balance right between personal and professional life?
- How do you remain true to yourself, when our working lives change so frequently and challenge us?
- What should you have in your 'toolkit' to ensure any personal conflict does not alter your very own being?

The answers I am afraid do not all lie in this chapter or in any one book. Yet, answers can lie within what you believe and seeking what works for you. Yet in this chapter there are some areas for you to consider when looking at what should be in your leadership 'kit bag'.

WHAT SORT OF A LEADER AM I?

I remember only too well an interview question once asked of me – *Can you describe your own leadership style*? Under pressure we often provide answers that we think may be what is being asked for, and then in hindsight wish we had expressed something differently. My immediate response quite simply was '*unique*'! In other words, we react, rather than respond, not always providing a meaningful answer. Exploring the impact of our actions – both mine and others – has led me to often be curious as to what makes a good leader. Here began my curiosity on leadership.

I, like many of you, do not fit into a box or into a single model of leadership. Neither do I believe I am a homogenous professional. I am professionally curious, with a leadership style that is characterised by a unique, adaptive nature and willingness to explore continuous development. If I do need to put myself into an approach, this aligns best with the concept of adaptive leadership, as described by Heifetz, Grashow, and Linsky (2009). They explain adaptive leadership as having the ability to adjust one's strategies in response to changing environments and challenges. Indeed, working in the NHS requires we must be adaptive and agile as the environment changes so frequently. To be able to respond to change, I believe that leaders must find ways of integrating their learning into everyday work experiences.

Yukl and Mahsud (2010) emphasise the significance of flexibility and learning if you wish to be an effective leader. There is a significant emphasis on successful leaders continuously evolving their approaches to meet the demands of their organisations and teams. Being aware of these needs and the ongoing development and adaptation that is required will ensure that leadership remains responsive and effective in diverse and dynamic contexts. For me, this adaptation and flexibility in my approach ensures I can function as an effective leader.

NAVIGATING THE COMPLEXITIES OF LEADERSHIP

In navigating the complexities of leadership, three core principles stand out as fundamental:

- *Authenticity* involves leading with a genuine sense of self.
- *Integrity* is the unwavering adherence to ethical principles.
- *Professionalism* encompasses the commitment to excellence and accountability in one's actions.

These three elements serve as the cornerstone of effective leadership and personal development. However, it should be noted that these are not mutually exclusive and therefore do not work in isolation. In essence the qualities possessed by leaders who are authentic, work with integrity, and remain professional are a core part of any effective leader, and one that is the bedrock of what makes me who I am.

AUTHENTICITY

Goffee and Jones (2005) emphasise that authentic leaders are true to their values and beliefs, fostering trust and loyalty among followers. Being authentic enables leaders to create a transparent and honest environment that encourages open communication and collaboration. It can be uncomfortable and difficult to work in this type of environment; however, high performing organisations and individuals will need to be able to achieve this level of transparency.

An authentic leader inspires loyalty and trust from others by consistently honouring commitments and keeping promises. Authentic leaders will also reinforce workers' emotional connection with their organisations and encourage them to increase individual creativity, which successively promotes better on-the-job performance. A demonstration of authentic leadership is through ensuring that you build a strong reputation for reliability and trustworthiness. Authenticity is the healthy alignment between internal values and beliefs and external behaviours. Authenticity comes from finding your style and your way of leading. Making decisions that reflect your ethics, values, and your personality.

One of the issues, however, with authentic leadership is that it brings our whole self into the professional space that we occupy. The problems associated with this is that there can be unconscious bias, which might temper our standing and interrupt our power to protect our teams, and so potentially compromise confidence. Although one may be open to the many ways a diverse workforce might effectively serve a community, it is difficult to support a fragile and exhausted team if you are feeling the same way.

Depending on where you are in your own personal leadership journey, this can be challenging, but navigating this is not impossible. If you know what you believe in and what your personal values are, others will more readily be able to place their trust in you – especially when they can see you are being true to yourself. Don't underestimate the fact that if you have that trust, it makes it possible to overcome challenges, and still get things done, as people know you have that level of authenticity, so there is trust in you, and you have trust in your staff to deliver.

Authentic leaders are individuals who are true to themselves and the principles that guide them as individuals. They are passionate about their work. They have a commitment to the organisation for whom they work and will often focus on the future ahead, ensuring everyone can find their place and be authentic themselves.

INTEGRITY

Covey (2004) asserts that integrity is the foundation of trust. This builds on the value of authenticity and is essential for effective leadership. Leaders who consistently demonstrate integrity build strong, trustworthy relationships, both personally and professionally whilst setting a positive example for their teams.

Integrity in leaders develops a strong sense of purpose and is about not shying away from the truth (which many people do not want to be confronted with) and ensuring an individual stands up for what is just and right. Making such a stance with integrity inspires and motivates others to follow their leader. Integrity is, in my opinion, not something that can be turned 'on' and 'off'. How others perceive leaders to be is not difficult. People can tell when someone is leading them on with falsehood, and you don't have to search hard to gauge the public's perception of leadership. Simply pick up any media coverage, such as a newspaper, or tune into an online news channel, and you'll be met with a barrage of stories expressing 'negative news' – which is all too often accompanied by widespread public frustration and commentary about how our 'leaders' are (mis)behaving.

A report by Professor Alan Renwick et al. (2022) identified that within politics, voters reported 'honesty' in leaders as being more important than delivery (71% versus 16%). The UK public want politicians who are honest, have integrity, and operate within the rules.

Integrity is revealed when observing actions more closely than relying on words. When someone's actions do not align with their words, it is a clear sign of a lack of integrity.

When thinking about my personal journey, integrity isn't just about whether someone is honest, but whether they strive to do the right thing in a variety of situations. Lacking integrity is often shown when someone prioritises their own interests above all else, such as seen in a dictatorship. It is something I consider when a person fails to even attempt to do the right thing. This often reveals a fundamental lack of integrity. Unfortunately, we will have all worked alongside an individual who lacks integrity. The issue, then, is how do you work with this?

Working with someone who shows a lack of integrity does not mean you should follow suit and start prioritising your needs over others. Being respectful of another individual and colleagues can be challenging; however, for effective teamwork, this is essential. When you disagree, focus on the problem or the process, rather than the individual. Keep feedback to things at the task level as much as possible, and do not focus on the personality, or how it makes you feel when they have let you down again by not completing what they said they would in good time. Essentially, provide feedback, stay respectful, open and honest, and remember that the working relationship with this person will not last forever.

PROFESSIONALISM

Professionalism is intrinsically related to good leadership. Hargreaves and Fullan (2015) highlight that professionalism involves a dedication to continual improvement and maintaining high standards. This commitment ensures that leaders not only achieve their goals but also inspire others to strive for excellence.

Leadership is not just about making decisions; it is about stewarding an organisation's values and instilling professionalism into the very fabric of the organisation by example. As a result of this, although it is not easy, it means treating your team with respect and trust, which, in turn, will earn their respect and trust.

Building trust with and among others requires good communication, cascading information between individuals, teams, and leaders is critical, as well as understanding what we're doing and why (through having a shared vision). When under pressure it's easy to forget, misunderstand, or just miss the relevance of something to be found in important communications. It is vitally important to revisit, revise and remind yourself and your teams of the vision and mission. For some, there is a need for many reminders. The repitiion of key message, can feel like deja vu for others, when these are having to be repeated at every meeting. People often only take notice when something has meaning or significance for them, so using varied ways of communicating is another good strategy for sharing those key messages.

By focusing on these three elements of authenticity, integrity, and professionalism, leaders can cultivate environments that are not only productive but also supportive and ethical. These principles provide a robust framework for navigating the challenges of leadership and achieving sustained success.

We need leaders with emotional intelligence and vision – leaders who are worth following because they embody the principles they preach and inspire confidence in their ability to lead with integrity. In simple terms, we want leaders who are visionary, principled, and truly deserving of our trust.

COMPASSION IN LEADERSHIP

Compassion is a crucial component of leadership. Goleman (1995) emphasises that emotional intelligence, which includes empathy, is vital for understanding and responding to the needs of others. Leaders who practice empathy can create supportive and collaborative environments, enhancing both team performance and individual satisfaction.

It is important to note that there are multiple influences on the capacity of an individual to be compassionate and to be able to offer this in their leadership. Specifically in healthcare this can relate to inadequate working conditions, poor leadership of self, role confusion, role conflicts, and excessive workloads.

It has been suggested that healthcare providers report not having time for 'compassion', due to the increase in regulation, burdening administration, and the need to reduce costs (Reiss 2015). The reasons offered remain true today, with evidence presented to the House of Commons health and social care committee in 2021 identifying that the discretionary effort offered by the workforce was not sustainable and workforce burnout was a significant issue. However, for leaders this can be a significant issue within the healthcare context. Leading a workforce successfully take its emotional toll on individuals.

Throughout my professional career there have been many influences on compassionate leadership that I have affected; however, a recent one has been through work undertaken with teams on the way in which they have delivered care.

Care with Kindness was developed because of several different data sets such as complaints, inpatient survey, FFT, etc. Where staff were, it was being reported care was 'rushed', or not 'kind', with little emphasis on an individualised, person-centred approaches. As a result, a programme was developed exploring the fundamentals of care delivery using learning approaches that encouraged staff to reflect on their practice and to encourage a safe psychological space for individuals to talk through care experiences that did not meet the Trust values of 'Fairness', 'Wellness', and 'Kindness'.

The design and delivery of the programme required clear leadership from ward to board underpinned by patient feedback and participation. Whilst the 'topics' may not change, working with people who have accessed and experienced our services does, which enhances positive outcomes for participants and develops understanding and learning from and in practice. Multimedia approaches to enable patient participation along with practical sessions with service users and voluntary groups, using interactive approaches to support learning in order that we can share and support some of the emotional 'turmoil' explored through reflection from practice.

Participants have remarked on the feeling of being in a group of like-minded staff who are able to 'carry on' – on a number of occasions staff had reported they felt they would leave their roles before the programme but now, having completed the Care with Kindness programme, are not looking to do so because they feel both enabled and empowered to question and deliver care that has kindness and compassion at its core.

This demonstrates how impactful leadership can be at all levels.

CASE STUDY

At a rare team away day, I was keen to invite each member of the team to share feedback on each other's progress, in an attempt to really get the team aware of each other's strengths and identified areas of development, so that we could then support each other to achieve those professional development goals.

As the team leader, I thought I had better take the first slot, role model the process, so I asked for feedback, focusing on my area of productivity. 'How can I ensure I remain responsive to you all? Particularly when sometimes I think I am really slowing down under the pressures of work, and therefore not keeping up to speed with all the demands being placed on us. Would you give me feedback on how you think I am doing in terms of my pace?'

At this request, the team looked aghast. I wondered at first, had I overstepped a boundary of professionalism here, in showing weakness, in revealing my self-doubt? But I held my breath and kept silent. I wanted to remain authentic and true to myself. What will they say? I braced myself for what was to come. Then one of them laughed, and several others joined in.

'Why are you laughing?' I asked. Again, my own self-doubt, imposter syndrome, and fear of rejection all swept through my mind.

'Really! You are worried you have slowed down?' they chimed. 'We wish you would slow down so we can keep up' was their unanimous response. More laughter ensued as relief spread throughout the team; they had all been having a similar experience.

One expressed in more detail with an example: 'I had four emails from you by the time I got in at 8 am. Please slow down, for your own sake, but also so I can get my responses back to you, in a meaningful way, as I want to give this my best as well.'

Another joined in: 'You are like a navy seal. You know, in the navy, they use dispersive leadership throughout the team, so they all know what to expect from each other when under pressure. It's in this podcast I have been listening to. I know that whatever you ask me to do, you have either already done this or would be able to do it yourself. That makes me feel I want to get work done, as I know you also want the best for me. Plus, you get the best out of us, as you encourage us all to do things we like, but to also try new areas to build new skills. This is a sign of a leader who is building a team and allowing us to be ourselves.'

PERSONAL JOURNEY OF LEADERSHIP

Unfortunately, we will not all have the experience outlined in the case study. Inevitably we will all have worked with the impact of poor leadership. Hopefully, you will have also experienced those with excellent leadership skills. The ability to offer a safe space, where you can listen to people and provide support to them, to then be able to make the right decision and move to the next stage of progression is critical.

In my professional life as a leader, I have helped colleagues through empowering them to make the best, informed decisions they needed to improve their work experience, career choices, and ultimately the care they offer, and to be confident to do the job they want, to be the best that they can be. West et al (2022) identified that staff who have influence over the decisions they make are likely to be better equipped to cope with work pressure because of the enhanced level of control they have over their decisions within the work environment, which is the basis of a positive experience for staff and for our patients, as this then cascades to the patients experiencing confident, happy staff.

LEADERSHIP CONTRIBUTES TO PERSONAL GROWTH

Kouzes and Posner (2017) argue that leadership is a journey of self-discovery. As leaders navigate challenges and opportunities, they develop personal resilience, self-awareness, and a deeper understanding of their personal values and goals. From personal experience, leading well and living well are reciprocal, in that each strengthens us. By leading with integrity, having and showing empathy, and a commitment to seeking balance in all of these, we can enhance our personal and professional lives. The journey of leadership is not just about achieving goals but also about becoming the best version of oneself. This leads to an enriching of both one's own life and the lives of others.

Throughout my career I have been fortunate to work with some amazing leaders. One of the most impactful leaders I worked with was someone from many years ago. As a student nurse I was given permission to learn and not be frightened to make mistakes. I was allowed to be 'me'; to learn how to be part of a team, and how every member of the team was important – whether it was the porter visiting the ward, the Health Care Assistant or the Consultant, we were all valued and all seen as an important part of what a successful team was made up of.

The Ward Sister showed me true leadership and promoted person-centred care, not only for our patients but to us as the entire multi-professional team. I have often reflected on the way in which the ward was led, and because everything we did mattered, the ward ran like clockwork. It was a wonderful example of a leader who acted with integrity, authenticity, and professionalism. Many years later when I met them again, they were just the same, a truly inspiring leader to the core.

Maintaining physical health is fundamental to overall well-being. There are other chapters in this book that explore the benefits of regular exercise, a balanced diet, and sufficient sleep, which are all critical components. Consistent physical activity can boost energy levels, improve mood, and reduce the risk of chronic diseases. Leaders who lead by example also engender a positive work-life balance and will increase a sense of well-being and likely enhance productivity.

It is not only physical health that indicates an individual's equilibrium but also their mental health, which is as important. Engaging in activities that reduce stress and promote relaxation, such as mindfulness, meditation, yoga can significantly impact mental well-being. There is a chapter on this too in the book to explore. Kabat-Zinn (2003) suggests that mindfulness practices can help individuals manage stress, enhance emotional regulation, and improve overall mental health, leaving you feeling ready to respond to people, rather than react. It is imperative that steps to achieve a better work-life balance is what matters. Human beings are inherently social creatures, and strong relationships are vital for well-being.

LEADING WITH KINDNESS AND COMPASSION

Kindness and compassion are important in values-driven leadership (Denney, 2020). It is this behaviour that is fundamental to caring for individuals we work with and who make up our teams. An integral part is always to question the challenges faced and acting to improve the working situation, accepting that this isn't easy in the volatile context we can find ourselves. All public sector services are politically and financially squeezed; the policy landscape can seem contradictory, and media scrutiny can be irresponsible, if not unkind, in their hunger for a good headline. Meeting performance and productivity expectations whilst promoting and protecting a diverse and sometimes depleted team can be fraught with emotional and intellectual contradictions alongside very real and pressing logistical tension.

Continuous learning and personal development contribute to a fulfilling life. Pursuing new hobbies, skills, or educational opportunities can keep the mind active and engaged. Dweck (2006) argues that adopting a growth mindset, which involves viewing challenges as opportunities for growth, can lead to greater resilience and long-term success.

A balanced approach that integrates physical health, mental and emotional well-being, strong social connections, lifelong learning, and self-compassion is necessary for a healthy work-life balance. Sounds easy, doesn't it? If we prioritise these practices, you can enhance your overall quality of life and sustain the energy needed to lead effectively.

I know only too well that cultivating meaningful relationships with family, friends, and colleagues can provide you with a circle of support that can help reduce stress and enhance overall happiness. In my professional life I have developed a short toolkit that has seen me through my leadership journey.

A LEADERSHIP 'TOOLKIT'

- Set clear boundaries to protect personal time and energy.
- Say no when necessary and avoid overcommitment, which can help prevent burnout.
- Treat yourself with kindness and understanding during times of failure or difficulty.

- Remember that everything presents an opportunity from which to learn.
- It's natural to get along with some people/colleagues more easily than others; there will be those you click with immediately and others with whom you struggle.
- Give yourself permission to have differences in the ways you relate.
- Leadership is not something you learn in a textbook; it is more about who you are and how you act and learning from what you have experienced.
- Good leadership takes time; however, keeping those we work 'for' and 'with' central to all that we do will ensure we make the right decisions
- Clear and effective communication is crucial and should be transparent and inclusive
- Create a supportive network of professional colleagues whose advice, guidance, and feedback you trust and differentiate this from those who might wish to put you down.
- Seek the time for self-compassion and self-care, as this will provide a strong foundation from which you can lead and role model others.
- Ask yourself, have you done the best you can in this situation? If you could look yourself in the mirror and say you have done the best you can, then that is a good indicator of success. If there is more to learn, then seek that out.

Leaders who give examples through their stories are more engaging. You influence the organisation's culture when you tell stories about what happened, about how a problem was solved, or about someone who did something notable. Narratives such as these can be far more powerful than a written summary.

I have not always had positive leadership role models; however, I have learnt as much from these negative or difficult situations as when I have had positive leadership experiences.

Here are a few more of my lessons learnt:

- It is not just about what you do, it's the difference you make.
- As a leader, it is the way you make others feel that will be remembered.
- Maintain professional curiosity and to feel comfortable to share all that you know.
- Maximising your own career ambitions is linked to your leadership ability.
- Being able to develop yourself into being a supportive leader plays a vital role in enhancing your individual skills and capabilities.
- As a leader you can provide guidance, resources, and opportunities for growth, you can empower your team members to reach their full potential,

and in turn if you receive this you will then be able to replicate it moving forward.

- Leaders who are ambitious are constantly developing themselves as well as their teams to do better.
- Set high standards and work tirelessly to achieve them.
- Mediocrity or complacency are not words that are associated with effective leaders, as they are always looking for ways to improve and to drive their organisations forward.

REFLECTION

What are some of the lessons you have learnt and noticed when working with either a great or an awful leader?

Whatever it is you take away from this chapter, it is about being true to who you are and to understand the impact you make.

Finally, remember that a strong leader does not have to be agreed with all the time. John Lydgate is attributed as saying 'You can please some of the people all the time, you can please all the people some of the time, but you cannot please all of the people all of the time.' However, always try to act with authenticity, integrity, professionalism, courage, curiosity, respect, compassion, and resilience. After all it's not about reading all the theory on leadership that makes for a great leader; it's about the reality of how you work alongside people, how you make people feel that makes for a strong, compassionate, authentic, kind leader who gets results.

FURTHER READING

Cardiff, S., Sanders, K., Webster, J. and Manly, K. (2020) *Guiding Lights Effective Workplace Cultures, IPDJ_1002_002.pdf* (last accessed 16th October 2022)

Holt-Lunstad, J., Smith, T. B. and Layton, J. B. (2010) Social Relationships and Mortality Risk: A Meta-analytic Review. *PLOS Medicine*, 7(7), e1000316.

Lawrence, J. (2023) Leading with love: Authenticity, vulnerability and compassion in contemporary. *HE Advance H.E* 06 Nov 2023

Mark LeBar. (2013) *The Value of Living Well*. Oxford University Press.

Neff, K. D. (2011) *Self-Compassion: Stop Beating Yourself Up and Leave Insecurity Behind*. William Morrow.

West, M., Bailey, S. and Williams, E. (2020) *The courage of compassion: Supporting nurses and midwives to deliver high-quality care*. The kings Fund The courage of compassion | The King's Fund Kingsfund.org.uk (last accessed 16th October 2022)

REFERENCES

Covey, S. R. (2004) *The 7 Habits of Highly Effective People: Powerful Lessons in Personal Change*. Free Press.

Denney, F. (2020). Compassion in Higher Education Leadership: Casualty or Companion During the Era of Coronavirus? *Johepal*, *1*(2), 41–47.

Dweck, C. S. (2006) *Mindset: The New Psychology of Success*. Random House.

Friedman, S. D. (2008) *Total Leadership: Be a Better Leader, Have a Richer Life*. Harvard Business Review Press.

Goffee, R. and Jones, G. (2005) *Why Should Anyone Be Led by You? What It Takes to Be an Authentic Leader*. Harvard Business Review Press.

Goleman, D. (1995) *Emotional Intelligence: Why It Can Matter More Than IQ*. Bantam Books.

Hargreaves, A. and Fullan, M. (2015). *Professional Capital: Transforming Teaching in Every School*. Teachers College Press.

Heifetz, R. A., Grashow, A. and Linsky, M. (2009) *The Practice of Adaptive Leadership: Tools and Tactics for Changing Your Organization and the World*. Harvard Business Review Press.

Kabat-Zinn, J. (2003). Mindfulness-Based Interventions in Context: Past, Present, and Future. *Clinical Psychology: Science and Practice*, 10(2), 144–156.

Kouzes, J. M. and Posner, B. Z. (2017) *The Leadership Challenge: How to Make Extraordinary Things Happen in Organizations*. Wiley.

Riess, H. (2015). The impact of clinical empathy on patients and clinicians: understanding empathy's side effects. *AJOB Neuroscience*, 6(3), 51–53.

Renwick, A., Lauderdale, B., Russell, M. and Cleaver, J. (2022) *What Kind of Democracy Do People Want? Results of a Survey of the UK Population First Report of the Democracy in the UK after Brexit* Project January 2022

West, T. H., Daher, P., Dawson, J. F., Lyubovnikova, J., Buttigieg, S. C. and West, M. A. (2022) The Relationship Between Leader Support, Staff Influence Over Decision Making, Work Pressure and Patient Satisfaction: A Cross-Sectional Analysis of NHS Datasets in England. *BMJ Open*, 12(2), e052778.

Yukl, G., and Mahsud, R. (2010) Why Flexible and Adaptive Leadership is Essential. *Consulting Psychology Journal: Practice and Research*, 62(2), 81–93.

Chapter 5

Well-being at work with some homework

Steve Green and Kate Roberts

INTRODUCTION

The psychological well-being of health and care staff is a key issue being faced by the National Health Service (NHS), and in other similar organisations providing health and social care globally. While the well-being of health and care staff has gained attention during the recent Covid-19 pandemic, this chapter discusses the importance of ongoing support for the psychological well-being for staff, as we navigate the recovery from the pandemic and beyond. During this chapter we will draw on the evidence base and our experience of developing a service to support staff well-being at a district general hospital in rural England to consider

- the importance of emotional support available to staff;
- the role of teams and managers in supporting staff psychological well-being;
- some techniques to try with your staff, and for yourself;
- how to check in and support your own work-related well-being; and
- spotting signs that you or a colleague may benefit from further evidence-based psychological support.

WELL-BEING AT WORK

Prior to the Covid-19 pandemic, NHS staff well-being was already highlighted as an area of concern due to high levels of work-related stress and burnout in the workforce, and the impact of this individually, financially, and for the running of safe and effective services (e.g. Health Education England, 2019). The Covid-19 pandemic subsequently placed healthcare workers under a sustained period of additional extreme pressures and uncertainty. During this time the NHS Staff

DOI: 10.4324/9781041057956-6

Survey showed an increase in staff feeling unwell with work-related stress over the past 12 months from 40.5 per cent in 2019 to 44.8 per cent in the 2022 survey (NHS Survey Coordination Centre, 2023). Preliminary data from the NHS Check study suggests that during the early months of the Covid-19 pandemic, 58.9 per cent of staff showed signs of a probable common mental health difficulty, and 30.2 per cent showed significant signs of post-traumatic stress disorder, based on responses to commonly used questionnaire measures of mental health (Lamb et al., 2021). In follow-up interviews, around one in five NHS staff members met diagnostic threshold for a mental health condition that could benefit from intervention (Pollitt and Pow, 2022). Stress and impact on mental health have also respectively been cited as the first and fourth most common reasons that NHS staff consider leaving the workforce (Weyman et al., 2023).

It is widely documented that staff health, well-being, and engagement is also associated with improved patient safety, patient experience, and effectiveness of patient care (Department of Health, 2009). Mental health conditions are also the most common reason for staff absences in the NHS, and are thought to have an associated cost of upwards of £3billion a year (NHS England and NHS Improvement, 2021), suggesting that improving staff well-being has the potential to lead to a significant positive impact on the cost of running services.

Overall, it is therefore evident that supporting staff's psychological well-being is important both for duty of care to individual employees, and the wider impact on services in terms of staff retention, patient outcomes, and cost effectiveness.

When discussing psychological well-being of the health and social care workforce, it is important to consider

- the direct impact of work on well-being. For example, the impact of having to make difficult decisions about a patient's care, or the impact of workplace bullying;
- the impact of wider life stressors and mental health on experiences at work. For example, if you are worried about a poorly relative at home, it may be more difficult to focus at work, or you may need workplace adaptations related to a longstanding mental health condition; and
- the interaction of and between the previous two. For example, during times of increased stress/responsibilities at home you may be more greatly impacted by work-related changes such as to scheduling of shifts.

Similarly, it is important to consider the different types of well-being interventions that can be implemented to support healthcare staff. One approach to understanding this is as three tiers of support, outlined by Kinman and Teoh (2018) based on a model developed by Firth-Cozens and Mowbray (2001):

- Primary interventions: preventative interventions that can be made to reduce causes of workplace stress (typically at an organisational level), in turn reducing the negative impact of work on staff well-being
- Secondary interventions: preventative interventions that focus on developing skills in staff members to feel more equipped to manage and respond to difficult work situations (for example, mindfulness or resilience training), that may in turn help reduce the impact of stressful events on individuals ongoing well-being
- Tertiary interventions: interventions to respond and help when a difficulty with psychological well-being already exists

This chapter draws on the experience of developing a staff support service at a district general hospital in a rural area of England. The service was developed in response to the Covid-19 pandemic, and has continued to be funded, evolving to meet the ongoing psychological needs of hospital staff. This service is psychology led and based physically on the hospital site. This allows input across all three tiers of intervention: advising on organisational well-being policy, running skills workshops for staff, and offering individual psychological therapy where needed. The rest of this chapter will describe the evidence that informed the development of the service, and learnings from practice, to offer advice for ways to support your own or your organisation's workplace well-being.

CASE STUDY

Being involved in my local hospital for over 20 years now, I have a real sense of pride in my work and where I work. It is a wonderful place, normally. But over the past few years, things have begun to get on top of me, as it were. I noticed that slowly, particularly since we all got moved about during Covid, that I have been less tolerant of staff who constantly moan about their shift patterns, or I avoid those who remind you of not having enough of this or that, or even that there is the wrong food in the canteen, or what really annoys me lately is when they remind me of the shocking price of a coffee that they manage to have time to pick up on the way to work. My jaw would be aching where I am desperately stopping myself snapping back at them.

At home, I just wanted to sleep all the time, but was never really feeling rested. My husband noticed I was easily wound up, whereas I used to be able to laugh, even when getting teased by the kids.

My manager also noticed a change in me. They asked me for a supervision session, which normally means going through a check list of, have you done this study day, have you kept your mandatory training up to date, but this time, they just sat and asked one question. 'How can I support you?'

This threw me, as I was not expecting it. To be offered something that normally was a phrase I used with my staff. We held each other's gaze for what felt like ages. Then the tears came. I hid my face in my hands at first. I was so embarrassed. Still nothing was said.

'I wonder if you would benefit from the staff support service? They have really helped me'; again I was shocked. My boss, the one person I thought had it all together, had sought help from the hospital staff support service.

'Well, if you think so', I answered glibly.

'Consider it a way to plug yourself back in, recharge yourself, rather like you do your mobile phone every night', they replied.

I left that meeting feeling churned up. Was I mentally ill? Was I being taken through a disciplinary process by being referred to the staff support service? Who else would find out? All these questions were running through my already busy head.

I did go. At first I had a chat with one of the team to find out more about what was on offer. They were so gentle with me and guided me through some of the things they could help me with. I immediately felt at ease. This was not about being disciplined at all. This was about me, and finding new ways of coping with all that a busy, hectic, draining working life brings.

I had several one-to-one sessions, took some reflective exercises home to work on, even some that involved asking things about myself with my family, and then later joined a resilience group.

Now I have people and places to really 'plug myself in', where I can reflect on what and how I take care of myself in this busy, hectic, chaotic world. It has also meant we are laughing with each other at home and with my colleagues at work again.

Thank you, staff support service. You have literally been a lifesaver for me, my work, and my family.

DEVELOPMENT OF THE STAFF SUPPORT HOSPITAL-BASED SERVICE

The Department of Clinical Health Psychology (DCHP) based at the district hospital was well established prior to the 2020 Covid-19 pandemic, with a team of psychologists primarily providing support to patients living with various physical health conditions. A limited service was also offered to provide staff psychological support, though the uptake was minimal with approximately 20 referrals received per year. As the staff pathway did not have any specific additional funding, the provision was also limited to the direct impact of work incidents on well-being (e.g. supporting staff members involved in traumatic medical incidents).

Following the government announcement on 23 March 2020 that the UK was going in to lockdown, and most routine hospital service provision was necessarily temporarily paused, the DCHP remained based on the hospital site (individual staff circumstances permitting) to provide psychological support for patients admitted to the hospital, and to provide psychological support to staff employed by the hospital who were either working at the hospital or having to redeploy to other services or roles. The service was available for clinical and non-clinical staff, and irrespective of whether or not they had direct contact with patients with Covid-19. The decision to offer staff support was based on guidance published in the immediate aftermath of the Covid-19 outbreak by the British Psychological Society (BPS) (British Psychological Society Covid-19 Staff Well-being Group, 2020), highlighting the potential psychologically traumatic impact of working in healthcare during a pandemic. The additional benefit of this provision being offered internally within the organisation is that as well as offering individual support for staff members, the team were able to offer advice to hospital leadership, training for managers to support preventative measures, and outreach to specific hospital areas at times of additional demand.

BRITISH PSYCHOLOGICAL SOCIETY COVID-19 GUIDANCE (2020)

The BPS guidance was produced to support the psychological well-being of healthcare staff during and after the Covid-19 pandemic. It was based on research arising from the Canadian SARS outbreak and from the earlier response to the Covid-19 outbreak in China, both of which identified healthcare staff experiencing increased levels of anger and irritability, higher levels of anxiety and low mood, increased alcohol drinking, smoking and eating, sleeping problems, and burnout. The aim of the guidance was to foster resilience, reduce burnout, and limit the risk of post-traumatic stress disorder (PTSD) amongst NHS and healthcare staff during and after the Covid-19 pandemic.

BPS guidance identified three psychological response phases mapping how healthcare staff needs were likely to vary across the course of the Covid-19 outbreak. The phases were described as Preparation Phase, dominated by anticipatory anxiety; the Active Phase, described as having two elements 'heroics/surge to solution' and 'disillusionment and exhaustion'; and the final Recovery phase, focussed on reflecting on the long-term psychological impacts of the pandemic and acknowledging that some staff could be at risk of chronic psychological difficulties, including (but not limited to) burnout and PTSD. The key recommendations for the Recovery phase (the phase that we are currently in, and therefore applicable to current NHS and healthcare staff psychological well-being needs) were the following (BPS, 2020, p. 5):

1. Allow space for taking stock, utilising trained practitioner psychologists to facilitate reflection and processing of experiences.
2. Organise active learning events that involve healthcare staff at all levels – feeding learning into future preparedness plans.
3. Organise thanks and rewards for everyday going above and beyond.
4. Needs assessment of staff – what did they find helpful, what ongoing input they would want now. If needed, increase your access to in-house Employee Well-being Services offering evidence-based psychological therapies.
5. Provide spaces for ongoing peer support.

IMPLEMENTATION OF GUIDANCE

The Clinical Health Psychology Department at the QEH based its response to the Covid-19 pandemic on the BPS guidelines outlined earlier, adapted and developed for the specific needs of the hospital. The underlying model of psychological

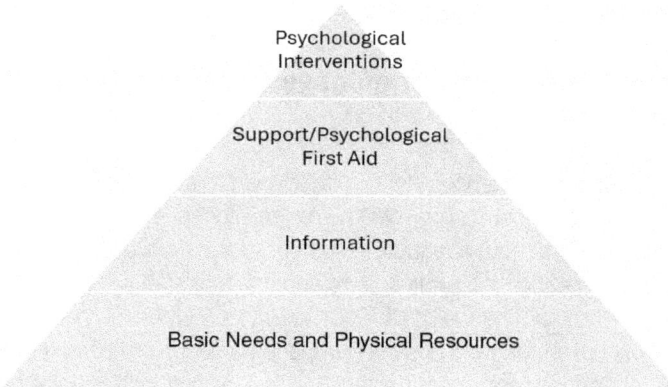

Figure 5.1 Stepped Psychological Response model (BPS, 2020, p. 3)

well-being support provision was the "Stepped Psychological Response" model proposed in the BPS guidelines (see Figure 5.1 subsequently).

The staff support service was initially provided from within the existing psychology staffing provision, with some redistribution of service from other specialties freed up due to Covid-19 restrictions. As the service developed, local charity funds were provided to increase availability of the service, which was then made substantial by the hospital in acknowledgement of the impact that the service had had on staff morale, retention, and well-being. Staff uptake of offered support was significant, rising from an average of 20 referrals received per year into the staff support service prior to 2019, to 352 referrals accepted in 2021, requiring 3168 individual appointments. Whilst the impact of the Covid-19 pandemic clearly affected referral rates, the numbers suggested that the change in service accessibility or provision had revealed an unmet need in hospital staff. Having a funded service specifically for staff also allowed the broadening of service provision, to also include supporting staff members where difficulties outside of work were negatively impacting their workplace well-being. To explore the impact of psychological support on staff well-being, retention, and patient outcomes, a research project is currently underway to identify and define the active ingredients of the support provided and to evaluate effectiveness.

The rest of this chapter introduces how staff well-being can be supported in healthcare services, using examples of how these recommendations were implemented at the hospital.

STAFF SUPPORT IN PRACTICE

Primary interventions – for managers, leaders, and organisations

As demonstrated by the Stepped Psychological Response model (Figure 5.1 earlier), support for staff emotional well-being ideally needs to start at an organisational level. Without adequate resource, information/training, and support to complete their jobs, it is understandable that staff will experience increased stress and poorer well-being. Furthermore, supportive management and colleagues have been found to positively impact mental health of staff (Kinman and Teoh, 2018). Therefore, fundamentally, individuals' psychological well-being within organisations can be considered dependent on support arising from within existing teams and support networks. Guidelines suggest that services should be careful of 'not rushing to psychology' to support individuals without this organisational level being addressed. Reflecting the importance of organisational support, the BPS Guidance (2020) comprised of ten key messages for NHS managers (p. 1–3):

1. Provide visible leadership.
2. Have a communication strategy.
3. Ensure consistent access to physical safety needs (e.g. personal protective equipment).
4. Ensure human connection and access to pre-existing peer support.
5. Provide psychological care to patients and families since this is key to staff well-being.
6. Normalise psychological responses.
7. Deliver formal psychological care in stepped ways.
8. Innovate to implement psychological care.
9. Come back to core NHS organisational and professional values in decision making.
10. Take care of yourself and pace yourself.

HOW THE SSS APPROACH HAS BEEN IMPLEMENTED [B]

Early in the development of the staff support service (SSS), to reflect the importance of 'visible leadership', a training programme for managers and team leaders was developed and rolled out. The hospital managers' training programme comprised of the BPS Guidance "Active Phase" advice for NHS leaders and managers (see earlier) and was delivered both face-to-face (with Covid-19 restrictions in place) and recorded for online access. The service also consults with the hospital leadership team on issues impacting workforce well-being, for example advising on supporting sleep in shift workers, access to rest areas, and the introduction of well-being passports (individualised plans for supporting staff members' well-being). Managers and team leaders who may be concerned about the emotional well-being of a staff member can also contact the staff support service clinicians if needed for advice about how best to offer support. The ability to offer this training and consultancy has been a notable benefit to the service being embedded within the organisation.

Individual well-being

As highlighted by both the stepped psychological response model (BPS, 2020), and Kinman and Teoh's (2018) tiers of support, in addition to the organisational changes, support should be available to individual staff members. The support available to individuals should be relative to their emotional needs at the time. Therefore, to best understand the type of support that may be most helpful for you, or for colleagues, it is first helpful to consider how your work-related well-being is at the moment. NHS Education for Scotland (2020) developed a helpful traffic light system (Table 5.2), which gives examples of physical, psychological, and social signs that you or someone else may be struggling with their well-being.

REFLECTIVE EXERCISE

Take a look through the earlier checklist and ask yourself these questions.

1. What's going well for you at the moment?
2. What's more difficult?
3. Overall, where would you say you are at right now – green, amber, or red?
4. How could you plan to regularly check in with your own well-being?
5. Go back to the case study example. If this was a member of your team, would you be able to know what is available to help them, based on your own experiences?

SECONDARY INTERVENTIONS: WHEN THINGS ARE 'GREEN' OR STARTING TO BECOME 'AMBER'

If things are generally going well with your well-being at the moment, the focus would be on trying to maintain this. One approach to this is focusing on the development of skills to improve our resilience. Resilience is not

Table 5.1 Common examples of signs that your well-being is at risk (NHS Education for Scotland, 2020)

Level of risk	Physical well-being	Psychological well-being	Social well-being
Green – no current risk	Usual levels of fitness and physical health Exercising as usual Sleeping well and feeling rested Eating and drinking as usual	Enjoying leisure activities Feeling well and focussed (while acknowledging variation in mood is natural) Feeling able to engage in things that would normally interest you	Feeling connected with colleagues Finding time and space to check in with each other Regular and fulfilling contact with family and/or friends
Amber – time to do something	Feeling more tired or 'run down' Doing less of the enjoyable activities Doing less of what brings meaning to life Changes to eating/drinking pattern	Feeling angry, stressed, or low in mood much of the time Finding it hard to focus Feeling overwhelmed at times Often thinking about difficult events that occurred during work	Reduced sense of connection with colleagues Reduced social contact Emotionally withdrawing from family and friends
Red – stop, take action	Disturbed sleep Exhausted Lethargic Significant changes in diet Increase in alcohol intake/substance misuse	Feeling overwhelmed or afraid much of the time Becoming angry at work and/or home Constantly thinking about difficult events at work	Isolating self Avoiding contact with colleagues Avoiding family and friends Anxiety about social contact or social activity (in person or virtually)

about having difficult days, or not experiencing emotional distress at these times, as that's normal and a very natural human reaction. Rather, in this context, resilience may be defined as our ability to bounce back following difficult experiences, including work-related stressors (Kunzler et al., 2020). This usually means looking after your own basic needs (e.g. sleep, nutrition), keeping connected to the things that give you a sense of meaning, keeping connected to the people in your life who are supportive (e.g. colleagues, friends, loved ones), and regularly checking in with our own thoughts and feelings. By noticing our thoughts and feelings, we are more able to catch sooner when things may be becoming difficult, and to develop skills to manage times of worry or self-criticism.

NHS Education for Scotland (2020) developed a helpful checklist of things that could be done in and outside of work to support your well-being. See Table 5.2 subsequently.

Table 5.2 Common examples of ways to preserve our well-being (NHS Education for Scotland, 2020)

Supporting your well-being	Physical well-being	Psychological well-being	Social well-being
At work	Give yourself permission to take breaks Eat and drink well Pace yourself	Take time to notice that there are things you can control and things you cannot Give your attention to the things you can change Understand your usual responses to stress – stress is a natural response Take brief 'mental' breaks when physical breaks are not possible – take a breath and reconnect with your body	Opportunities for regular check-in with colleagues Work with a buddy where possible Maintain connection with outside supports during breaks

(Continued)

Table 5.2 (Continued)

Supporting your well-being	Physical well-being	Psychological well-being	Social well-being
On leaving work	Do a physical check: Am I ok? What do I need to do to look after myself now? Who can I speak to if I need anything?	Reflect on the day Acknowledge difficult events and let them go Acknowledge 3 things that went well Switch attention to going home Rest and recharge	Check in with colleagues: "Are you ok?" Connect with colleagues to review the day if that feels helpful to you
At home	Balance – plan activities that you know support you to relax and unwind Prioritise rest, eating, and some physical exercise Have a routine to wind down before bed	Awareness – notice the impact of the day Develop and use a wind-down routine to disconnect from work Take time to consciously choose to switch focus from work to home	Connection – stay connected with the people and activities that are important to you Remind yourself of your values. Why do you do what you do? Why is it important to you?

A GROUP RESILIENCE PROGRAM

In addition to widely available general advice and resources (like the earlier checklist), a colleague in the staff support service developed a group resilience program for staff members (Cassidy, unpublished). This group was informed by earlier work by Baker et al. (2021). The group is run as a four-part workshop based on cognitive behaviour therapy (CBT), and topics include

- introducing resilience,
- understanding emotional reactions to a difficult experience,

- noticing and managing unhelpful thoughts,
- connecting to sense of purpose/meaning,
- relaxation exercises, and
- reflections on personal strengths.

Staff members can access this program through the psychology department, or requests for the group to be run for a specific team may be made by managers/ team leaders. This has widened the preventative support available for hospital staff.

REFLECTION

Spend some time looking through the earlier recommendations. Consider the following.

1. What are you already doing that helps your well-being?
2. What is an area you would like to improve?

When you have done this, try setting for yourself a goal towards improving your self-care. This is most likely to be helpful if you set a goal that is small and achievable, and you make a clear plan for how and when to make the change.

TERTIARY INTERVENTIONS: WHEN THINGS ARE 'AMBER' OR 'RED' [B]

If when you looked at the traffic lights (Table 5.1 earlier) you felt you are currently in the 'red' zone, or if you are feeling stuck in 'amber', this would be a sign that seeking some individual evidence-based psychological support would be helpful. If you are not sure what's available to you locally, the first step would be to reach out to your manager, occupational health, or your GP, whoever you feel most comfortable to approach, as they should be able to direct you to the services that are available to you locally.

INTRODUCING PSYCHOLOGICAL FIRST-AIDERS

The staff support service is based on the stepped care model, recognising the 'not rush to psychology' advice. However, the service also recognised the importance of reducing barriers to accessing support when needed. During the initial set-up of the service, several means of accessing support were therefore introduced, supported by 'advertising' in the form of posters placed around the hospital, a lanyard card, desktop screensavers, and working closely with the hospital communications department. These included

- a dedicated phone support line;
- dedicated "drop in" spaces in hospital grounds (staffed between 6 am and 9 pm to allow access during shift changes for night staff);
- ward-based drop-ins;
- education and reflection groups; and
- individual psychological therapy (accepting self-referrals or referrals from managers or occupational health with the staff member's consent).

Over time, to provide support to the growing referrals to the SSS team, psychological first aid training was delivered to volunteer hospital staff who were supported by their managers to allocate time to the role. The training was derived from World Health Organization et al. (2011) 'Psychological First Aid: A guide for field workers' and NHS Education for Scotland (2020). The training was provided for 35 hospital staff supported with monthly supervision and access to the staff support psychology team outside of this for escalation of support if required. The role comprised of learning to identify signs of emotional distress, how to support a person in immediate need, and to signpost for further support if required. Being NHS staff, psychological first aiders were already embedded within staff teams and therefore able to provide a 'first line' of support if staff felt willing and able to approach the psychological first aiders, and thus complemented the 'ease of access' philosophy, though first aiders could be contacted directly from any staff team by any staff member. The psychological first aid approach continues to provide ongoing support and has aided a cultural change of embedding psychological well-being within he hospital.

Since the introduction of the psychological first aiders, and moving to the recovery phase of the pandemic, the routine phone line and drop-in support offered by the psychology department were stopped. However, ongoing open access to individual assessment and therapy remains, with onwards referral to specialist services where needed post-assessment. Education and reflective groups also continue, and specific outreach support to certain staff groups/hospital areas is offered when a need is highlighted. This has allowed a more sustainable stepped care approach to be taken with the available resource, and the department continues to benefit from the increased awareness within the workforce developed during the initial period of increased outreach.

CONCLUSION

There is currently high levels of stress and mental health difficulties amongst the healthcare workforce. Better supporting healthcare staff is in the best interests of organisations for duty of care to employees, staff retention, patient outcomes, and financial efficiency. To best support staff well-being, intervention is needed at both an organisational and individual level, with individual support proportionate to current emotional needs. This chapter provides an example of how a within-organisation psychology-led staff support service can be used to support the emotional well-being of staff, through the provision of training and consultation to managers and leaders, the ongoing support and training for individuals who can provide first line on the ground emotional support, as well as offering direct evidence-based psychological support to staff members when needed.

FURTHER READING

- Health Line: How to keep work stress from taking over your life. www.healthline.com/health/work-stress
- Mindtools: Creating a health workplace www.mindtools.com/a299wr1/creating-a-healthy-workplace
- NHS Helpline: Stress at work www.nhs.uk/mental-health/feelings-symptoms-behaviours/feelings-and-symptoms/stress/

REFERENCES

Baker, F., Baker, K. and Burrell, J. (2021) Introducing the skills-based model of personal resilience: Drawing on content and process factors to build resilience in the workplace. *Occupational and Organizational Psychology*, 94(2), pp. 458–481.

British Psychological Society Covid-19 Staff Wellbeing Group. (2020) *The psychological needs of healthcare staff as a result of the Coronavirus pandemic*. Leicester, British Psychological Society.

Cassidy, C (2023) *How to be resilient: An evidence-based approach to cultivating resilience*. Unpublished.

Department of Health. (2009) *NHS health and well-being*. Final Report. London, Department of Health

Firth-Cozens, J. and Mowbray, D. (2001). Leadership and the quality of care. *BMJ Quality & Safety*, 10, pp. ii3–ii7.

Health Education England. (2019) *NHS staff and learners' mental wellbeing commission*. Birmingham, Health Education England.

Kinman, G. and Teoh, K. (2018) *What could make a difference to the mental health of UK doctors? A review of the research evidence*. [Online] Available at: www.som.org.uk/sites/som.org.uk/files/What_could_make_a_difference_to_the_mental_health_of_UK_doctors_LTF_SOM.pdf [Accessed 30 July 2024]

Kunzler, A., Helmreice, I., Chmitorz, A., König, J., Binder, H., Wessa, M. and Lieb, K. (2020) Psychological inteventions to foster resilience in healthcare professionals. *Cochrane Database of Systematic Reviews*. [Online] Available at: https://doi.org/10.1002/14651858.CD012527.pub2

Lamb, D, Gnanapragasam, S, Greenberg, N, Bhundia, R., Carr, E., Hotopf, M., Razavi, R., Raine, R., Cross, S., Dewar, A., Docherty, M., Dorrington, S., Hatch, S., Wilson-Jones, C., Leightley, D., Madan, I., Marlow, S., McMullen, I., Rafferty, A.M., Parsons, M., Polling, C., Serfioti, D., Gaunt, H., Aitken, P., Morris-Bone, J., Simela, C., French, V., Harris, R., Stevelink, S.A.M. and Wessely, S. (2021) Psychosocial impact of the COVID-19 pandemic on 4378 UK healthcare workers and ancillary staff: Initial baseline data from a cohort study collected during the first wave of the pandemic. *Occupational and Environmental Medicine*, 78, pp. 801–808.

NHS Education for Scotland. (2020) *Wellbeing planning tool*. Edinburgh, NHS Education for Scotland. Available at: https://learn.nes.nhs.scot/30741/psychosocial-mental-health-and-wellbeing-support/taking-care-of-myself/wellbeing-planning-tool [Accessed 30 July 2024]

NHS England and NHS Improvement. (2021) *NHS health and wellbeing framework: elements of health and wellbeing*. Available at: https://www.england.nhs.uk/publication/nhs-health-and-wellbeing-framework [Accessed 30 July 2024]

NHS Survey Coordination Centre. (2023) *NHS staff survey 2022: National results briefing*. Oxford, NHS Staff Survey Coordination Centre.

Pollitt, A. and Pow, R. (2022). *Supporting the mental health of NHS staff as part of post-pandemic recovery*. London, NHS Check and The Policy Institute at King's College London.

Weyman, A., Glendinning, R., O'Hara, R., Coster, J., Roy, D. and Nolan, P. (2023). Should I stay or should I go. *NHS staff retention in the post COVID-19 world: challenges and prospects-IRR report*. In.: University of Bath.

World Health Organization et al. (2011). *Psychological first aid: Guide for field workers*. Geneva, WHO.

Chapter 6

Social encounters at work

Sharing is indeed caring

*Georgia Panagiotaki, Susanne Lindqvist
and Joel Owen*

INTRODUCTION

Caring for others is hard. It takes a lot of effort and energy. Doing it well also requires that we pay attention to ourselves. If you work in health and social care, you will have had days when you felt exhausted, overwhelmed or out of your depth. For years, the pressure on health and social care staff has increased, so much so that a growing number of people are leaving the profession. Those who once thought of joining the health and social care workforce now hesitate. The central idea of this chapter is that sharing our experiences with others and discussing how we feel about our work is an important way of looking after ourselves, our colleagues and, ultimately, our patients. Let us lead you through an approach to work that values sharing emotions, promotes openness and restores the central place that humanity has in the caring professions. In doing so, we can help to attract the future health and social care workforce and nurture the relationships and well-being of its members. Let us bring back hope and share good practices that really work.

To thrive, whether as students or as trained clinicians, people need to be equipped to learn and work *together*. This needs to be nurtured throughout each person's professional education and career, so that meaningful social encounters across different professions becomes an enriching experience. Working openly in this way can help bridge gaps, capture opportunities and horizon scan to explore future solutions whilst considering new ways of working, together. By learning more about what our colleagues think and how that influences what they do,

DOI: 10.4324/9781041057956-7

we become more open to recognising that our similarities and differences are all important in getting it right for the patient's personalised care. This in turn increases our compassion, understanding and connectedness with others. Sharing is indeed a way of caring.

Professional training represents a critical moment, a point at which many of the attitudes, practices and beliefs that shape and inform one's career are being formed or re-formed. So, how can we embed this intuitive way of learning and working into the curricula during individuals' education, training and lifelong careers? More than ever before, we need to embrace caring as a mindset to inspire and empower each other to share knowledge, thoughts and feelings about matters that affect us in our working lives. Importantly, when we help create safe environments that allow people to share, listen and reflect, it can offer the much-needed reflective time that can sustain and improve our working lives. This compassionate approach is at the very core of Interprofessional Schwartz Rounds, and the interpersonal care that these facilitated groups promote.

WHAT ARE SCHWARTZ ROUNDS?

Rounds (as they are known for short) are the legacy of health attorney Ken Schwartz, who was diagnosed at a young age with terminal lung cancer. What he noticed and shared with others during his treatment was that the small acts of kindness he received from his caregivers made the biggest difference to his harrowing experience, and 'made the unbearable bearable'. Quiet acts of humanity, such as a gentle touch or reassuring word, felt more healing than the radiation or chemotherapy treatments promising hope of a cure. What Ken Schwartz also acknowledged was that professionals can deliver compassionate and high-quality care only if they themselves feel emotionally supported and cared for by their organisation. Before he died, he left a legacy for the establishment of the Schwartz Center Rounds in Boston, United States (USA), to help foster compassion in healthcare.

Schwartz Rounds were established in the 1990s in the USA and brought to the United Kingdom (UK) by the Point of Care Foundation (PoCF), a non-profitable organisation focusing on humanising healthcare and holding the license to run Rounds in the UK. Rounds provide an inclusive, interprofessional, structured space for facilitated reflection, in which clinical and non-clinical staff come together to discuss the emotional and social nature of working in healthcare. Rounds are not intended to solve clinical problems. Instead, they offer a safe space to discuss the challenges and rewards of clinical work.

REFLECTION

- If you are not familiar with Schwartz Rounds, you can use this chapter to find out how they work and what they offer. The end of the chapter explains how to find and watch an edited video of a Schwartz Round, so you can get a feel for how they work.
- Perhaps you have Schwartz Rounds in your organisation? If you do, we invite you to use this chapter as a prompt to attend an upcoming Round.
- Take a look at the further reading and materials we have provided at the end of this chapter to further stimulate your interest.

Rounds differ from more traditional staff forums such as grand rounds or Balint groups. They focus on participants' experiences, rather than the clinical aspects of patient care, and are open to all members of an organisation, including non-clinical staff. Rounds are not designed to offer clinical supervision, nor a forum for debriefing following stressful or traumatic clinical events. Their central function is to allow participants across different disciplines to move away from their usual position of urgent action and problem solving, to an hour of quiet reflection, stillness and open sharing (Atkins et al., 2023; Wren, 2016). In this sense, Rounds offer a counter-cultural space, where participants role model vulnerability and show generosity towards others and self (Maben & Taylor, 2021).

When Rounds are delivered in person, food is available and shared amongst participants before the storytelling begins. Sharing food is an important part of this practice. It is a symbolic act of being physically and psychologically nourished.

Each Round lasts one hour and centres around a topic along the lines of 'a patient I'll never forget', 'a day I made a difference', or 'in at the deep end'. Topics are usually chosen in advance by a Schwartz Round steering group whose role is to plan, deliver, promote and evaluate Rounds in their organisation. To ensure attendees feel they are in a safe environment, two trained facilitators – also members of the steering group – are present at each Round. Their role is to introduce three or four pre-chosen storytellers who tell a short and uninterrupted story on an agreed topic. These stories have been prepared carefully between storytellers and facilitators to ensure the psychological safety of the storytelling. Facilitators are only permitted to take on this role once they have completed a two-day bespoke training delivered by the Point of Care Foundation.

Following the stories, members of the audience are invited to share their own thoughts on what they have heard. Facilitators help the group to contain strong emotions that can arise from these discussions (such as anger, fear or grief) and create a space where members can reflect openly, feel heard and have the necessary time to sit with their emotions. Recognising the importance of supporting those who share as well as those who listen (Winn & Lindqvist, 2019), support is also offered to the storytellers who may not have shared their stories in this way before.

Schwartz Rounds are predicated on the 'power of storytelling' (Irvine et al., 2023) and its potential to support the emotional well-being of health practitioners who undertake complex interpersonal work under stressful conditions. The opportunity for storytellers to prepare their stories in dialogue with facilitators, and to narrate them within a Round of engaged listeners, has the potential to be therapeutic for those individuals. Equally, hearing others' stories can help affirm the idea that health and social care professionals are 'also human' (Ng et al., 2022) and have emotional responses to the work they do. Indeed, there is increasing evidence across the world that Rounds have the capacity to support the emotional self-care of health and social care practitioners.

Research evidence shows that regular attendance of Rounds is associated with significant improvements in staff psychological well-being and positive changes in patient care delivery. Although their impact takes some time to develop, Rounds have been shown to reduce professional hierarchies, improve communication between colleagues and decrease work stress and compassion fatigue (PoCF, 2022). They can increase empathy and compassion towards patients and colleagues and reduce feelings of isolation (Maben et al., 2018; Maben & Taylor, 2021). We will explore this further when meeting Alex in the subsequent case study.

CASE STUDY

Alex is a 27-year-old nursing student approaching the end of their course. They have always considered themselves to be a compassionate person, and someone who knew from early on that they wanted to work in a caring profession. Alex experienced the early years of their course as fast-paced and exciting, when they were soaking up a wealth of new knowledge and developing a range of new competencies. In recent months, however, the weight of their future role as a qualified nurse has begun to weigh heavily on them, and they report frequently feeling out of their depth and overwhelmed by the responsibility of their future role.

Alex has found it difficult to stay motivated and engaged at work and in study. They often feel emotionally exhausted. Alex has kept these feelings from friends and colleagues, worried that they will be misinterpreted as signs of poor coping. The longer they feel like this, the more they question the values that brought them into nursing in the first place and whether they can ever be a good nurse. When looking at the future, Alex wonders whether they will ever be able to qualify and manage the expected responsibility associated with looking after patients.

On the wards and in the classroom, Alex sees peers facing similar challenges and wonders how everyone seems to manage. Supervisors appear to be untouchable, impervious somehow to the stressors of the work. The academic staff demonstrate an almost unattainable ideal of competence. Gradually, Alex is starting to waver about their dream of becoming a nurse and starts thinking about dropping out and wondering if they should change career paths.

Alex spotted a poster about an Interprofessional Schwartz Round being run by faculty at their university. They decide to attend out of curiosity. Knowing little about what to expect, Alex sat quietly at the back of the room and listened to three storytellers talking about 'a day I'll never forget'.

Each storyteller recounts a significant day in their work as healthcare professionals, covering the highs, the lows and the expansive middle ground in between. The complicated combination of anxiety and excitement felt by a trainee doctor on the first day of their medical training, the still-present sadness described by a senior paramedic the first time they encountered death at work and the exhausted tears of pride cried by a ward manager after a family member had thanked them for the way they had looked after their elderly mother. All these stories resonated forcefully with Alex. Each story seemed to capture the deeply human nature of clinical work, revealing both the resilience and fragility that defines so much of our experiences, as people and professionals.

Alex left the Round that day feeling lighter than they had done for many weeks. They felt they had shared more in common with the storytellers than they would have imagined, which made Alex feel more connected to those around them. As such, they had lost many of the feelings of being alone with their feelings. The distant ideals that colleagues had once represented were challenged in a way that revealed a more grounded, connected and realisable vision of working in healthcare. Though Alex had listened without contributing during the Round, they felt empowered to speak more openly about their work, and to sit more comfortably with the complex interplay of emotions that defined their experience of working in healthcare.

LEARNING FROM ALEX'S STORY: A REFLECTIVE ACTIVITY

- Take a moment to reflect on whether Alex's story resonates with your own experience, or that of a colleague or peer. For example, think of a time in your own training or work life when you felt overwhelmed by the responsibility of the role and the challenge of doing it well. Alternatively, think of a time that is closely connected to feelings of satisfaction, pride or enjoyment.
- Using a reflective model such as Driscoll's (2007) can help to define specific areas of reflection. Driscoll's model is centred around answering three key questions in relation to your experience: *What? So what? Now what?*
- **What?:** Describe the experience (e.g. in which you felt overwhelmed, or particularly proud). What happened?
- **So what?:** What did you think and feel? How much did you discuss your feelings with others? What did it feel like to share good or bad times with others? If you didn't share, what may be the reason? What needs to happen at work for you to feel better able to share?
- **Now what?:** What have you learned from this experience? What inspiration can you take? What might you do differently (or more of) going forward?

Another model you can use in this activity is Gibb's (1998) reflective cycle. It focuses on six areas around an experience you are reflecting on:

The next section looks in more detail at Schwartz Rounds in higher education, where they have recently been integrated as an innovative way of supporting

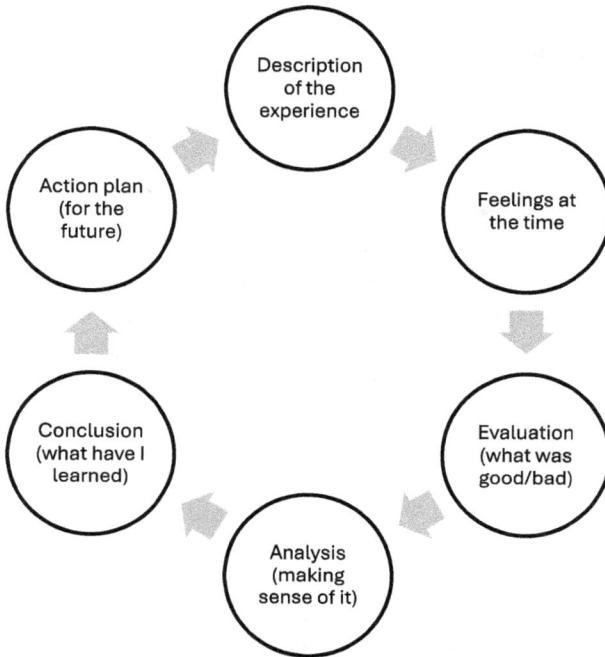

Figure 6.1 Reflective cycle adapted from Gibbs (1998)

health professional students' reflective practice, interprofessional learning and compassionate care.

Schwartz rounds in higher education

Whilst at university (college or higher education), health and social care learners accrue a wealth of clinical skills and competencies required to work as part of the modern workforce. Yet, too many enter their professional field feeling under-equipped to manage the emotional and human vulnerabilities that form an integral part of their roles.

Schwartz Rounds have run successfully in practice settings since they were brought to the UK by the PoCF in 2009. As seen in the case study earlier, they are now also becoming an impactful source for learners such as Alex, whilst preparing for their future roles. Rounds provide an ideal opportunity to introduce health and social care learners to the attitudes and behaviours of compassion, openness and self-care that are central to a fulfilling career. By embedding Rounds into curricula and encouraging a focus on the human side of caring, educators can further support the health, well-being and sustainability of the emerging workforce.

In line with research on the effectiveness of Rounds in clinical settings, growing evidence suggests that they can support health and social care students in powerful ways (Hamilton et al., 2023). They offer a safe space for dialogue between participants that helps normalise strong emotions arising from learners' education. They enable learners to appreciate the work that other health professionals do as part of the wider system. Meeting in this way allows for impactful interprofessional insights about the different roles involved in patient care. Importantly, Rounds can equip students with a potentially career-long ability to think and talk about how they feel in the context of their work and training (Clancy et al., 2020; Zervos & Gishen, 2019).

Given that an increasing number of higher education institutions are now embedding Rounds in their curricula, we invite you to explore whether they are offered in your institution and to consider getting involved as a participant, storyteller or Rounds ambassador. Your involvement will be valuable to others, and a way of supporting your own well-being. Just as we saw in the case of Alex, Rounds can be a powerful medium for supporting well-being and enhancing a feeling of connection during training.

Our research on the impact of interprofessional Rounds on health and social care students at the University of East Anglia (Zile et al., 2024) suggests that attendees benefit from participating in this form of reflective practice. Students and staff who have responded to our evaluation and interview questions tell us that Rounds are emotive and powerful. Participants rate the Rounds as 'excellent' or 'exceptional'. One hundred per cent of student attendees say that hearing others talk about their personal feelings in the context of their work is helpful to them. Students attend the Rounds out of curiosity and because it helps them to keep engaged in their course. Because of their experiences in previous Rounds, around 80 per cent of our student attendees think Rounds should be introduced into their curriculum, and over 85 per cent report that Rounds have offered them insight and knowledge that equips them for clinical practice. Many feel that Rounds offer a safe space for reflection that deepens their compassion and empathy.

Here are some direct quotes from students who have taken part in one or more interprofessional Schwartz Rounds at UEA during 2023–24:

I have attended previous Rounds and have always found them to be a very thought provoking, powerful experience which helps drive home the human side of healthcare.

I thought the story tellers were brave discussing their fears, feelings and experiences – and that by doing this they created a safe space for others to share. Thank you to all!

It deepened my compassion and empathy toward colleagues across the various disciplines in healthcare. . . . It felt empowering, validating, and it consolidated my personal values in relation to my professional responsibilities.

Looking at the published literature and our own findings, evidence indicates that Schwartz Rounds can help create a safe space for staff and students to share how they feel and to discuss things they experience that may be challenging to carry alone. Introducing Rounds from the beginning of students' education and throughout professionals' careers provides a sense of stability and community of practice that can help foster a culture of sharing. As discussed by Canzan and Colleagues (2022), role modelling is important when it comes to supporting students as they face fears and doubts about their career choice. Hence, even if you do not feel you 'need it', you may be the one who can help someone who does. It may be your story that chimes with someone like Alex. This resonates with the NHS People Promise (2024) that pledges to improve the workplace for staff.

THE CHALLENGES AND REWARDS OF WORKING AND TRAINING IN THE MODERN HEALTHCARE WORKFORCE

A well-developed body of literature indicates that working in the health and social care workforce brings with it both challenges and rewards. Clinicians across a range of professions frequently report that their work is associated with meaning and purpose (Flanagan et al., 2019; Russo-Netzer et al., 2020), personal values (Rider et al., 2014) and a sense of enjoyment, interest and satisfaction (Jones & Green, 2006). However, professionals in these fields also frequently report high levels of burnout, stress and poor mental health (Morse et al., 2012; Simionato & Simpson, 2018). Some researchers have suggested that work in this field presents several unique challenges that increase vulnerability to burnout (Maslach & Leiter, 2016). In the last few years, the pressures applied to the modern healthcare workforce following Covid-19 and the systemic and structural challenges currently facing the NHS have also amplified this problem (Hill et al., 2022).

In preparing our future workforce, we often see how learners arrive filled with enthusiasm, keen to learn and excited to be entering a field of work they have often long aspired to. Whilst for many an exciting career rich in the rewards and realities of this work follows, too often, the stresses experienced during their course leads to dropout, disillusionment or ill-health. Sadly, in turn, these experiences may feed into their qualified careers if not dealt with in a timely and appropriate fashion. Canzan et al. (2022) reported findings of students becoming disillusioned, describing the need for them to come together with other peers to overcome anxieties and share experiences so that they can re-gain faith that their chosen professional path is right for them.

We continue to hear that the NHS workforce is 'on its knees', yet funding continues to be constrained, and vacancy freezes are introduced to mitigate cost. This is impacting on patient care and our remaining staff, many of whom are experiencing burnout. The House of Commons Health and Social Care Committee report (2021) highlights staff burnout and resilience and makes recommendations for how to facilitate well-being and promote compassionate leadership in healthcare. In an article by NHS employers (2024), the need for preventative action for the fostering of a compassionate culture at work is also emphasised. Senior leaders can be impactful role models in supporting and nurturing a compassionate culture in their organisations, and Schwartz Rounds offer huge potential in this regard. By connecting staff from across all career stages and within multiple professions, Rounds offer a valuable format for supporting the development of a compassionate working culture that extends across the whole of an organisation. With the support and culture that can flow from Rounds, students like Alex can be supported to experience health and social care as a meaningful, realisable and fulfilling career.

In this chapter we have drawn on published literature and our own experience running Interprofessional Schwartz Rounds at UEA to present Rounds as an example of an intervention that can support well-being and compassion, whilst nurturing a sense of purpose and value amongst those studying and working in healthcare. If you are interested in this form of reflective practice, finding out more about what is offered in your organisation may be a helpful first step. A now large and ever-growing number of organisations (both within healthcare and higher education) run Rounds, so we encourage you to look into what is available where you work or study. If you can find Rounds running nearby, we hope this chapter inspires you to attend. To help readers who might be interested in setting up or getting involved with Rounds at their organisation, we've thought carefully about things which have helped or hindered us in establishing and running Rounds where we work, in the hope this can be of help to others.

Firstly, organisational buy-in is paramount. Rounds can offer a significant range of benefits, but they do require an investment of time and resource, both to run the Rounds themselves and to train facilitators in a way that ensures they can be run with fidelity. A committed Steering Group of invested individuals is key to helping drive this, so a good place to start may be to seek out others in your organisation with an interest in this area. Attendance at Rounds can also be challenging for professionals and trainees who have busy schedules, so varying the time and format (e.g. face-to-face vs online) can help to reach the widest range of people possible. Once people attend, it's also important to monitor feedback and to use trained facilitators to gauge the extent different themes resonate with audiences, so that future Rounds can be designed in a way to capitalise on what has worked best so far. To encourage the interprofessional aspect, and so that we can help equip learners to thrive as part of a collaborative health and social care workforce, some of the universities running Rounds are also linked to the UK Centre for Interprofessional Education (CAIPE).

FACILITATORS AND BARRIERS IN SETTING UP AND RUNNING SCHWARTZ ROUNDS

Table 6.1 Barriers and facilitators identified from introducing interprofessional Schwartz Rounds in the higher education setting

Barriers	Facilitators
Don't know where to even start or who to contact	You can contact any of the authors of this chapter or a Schwartz Round facilitator in your workplace, or contact Point of Care, and someone may be able to help.
Time and commitment (Rounds are resource intensive).	An invested and engaged steering group that role-model interprofessional working.
One cannot conduct Schwartz Rounds without trained facilitators and a contract with PoCF, which ensures quality but can be seen as expensive.	Fidelity to the UK Schwartz Rounds model.
Without continued support, sustainability may become an issue, particularly during difficult financial climate.	Teams supported by their organisation.

(Continued)

Table 6.1 (Continued)

Barriers	Facilitators
Not everyone is on board yet, and there is a risk that even good initiatives can disappear without buy-in across the organisation.	National organisations (PoCF) or professional regulatory bodies (e.g. HCPC) being explicit about the benefits.
Finding a rounded panel can become challenging over time.	Interprofessional panel of story tellers helps to resonate with broad potential audiences.
Students' timetables and incorporating it into students' curricula can be challenging.	Vary the timing and offer, face-to-face and online. Rather than making it compulsory, keep it voluntary, but try encourage involvement and curiosity; and also share good experiences where students and staff feel it made a difference to them.
Theme not 'hitting the right note', which makes it difficult for the audience to relate.	Trained facilitators will skilfully help make sure this does not happen and take onboard feedback so that future themes can be enhanced.
Sustainability	Renewal of steering group members to ensure not all leave at the same time but that the good practice can be transferred, and that succession planning is embraced.

CONCLUSION

The central idea of this chapter has been that sharing is caring. When we share with colleagues, peers, fellow learners and supervisors, we connect with each other and encourage an attitude of openness to experience. Importantly, some research indicates that oversharing, or unhelpful venting of emotions, can be unproductive and associated with poor well-being. Against this, Schwartz Rounds offer a safe and effective forum for facilitating a form of sharing that is helpful and contained. It was this sentiment of sharing that resonated with and supported Alex in the case study earlier. It is also this sentiment that we hope you can take away from this chapter.

Sharing in the way described in this chapter helps to model vulnerability and emphasise the deeply human nature of caring work, something we believe is critical for supporting the well-being of the workforce and the people that it serves. Working in health and social care involves a dichotomy of emotive feelings that are regularly enriching and uplifting yet frequently challenging. Caring for others is hard, and caring for ourselves is sometimes even harder. It is therefore important to share moments of pain, success, loss and gain. By providing a safe space to think and reflect together and talk openly about the ups and the downs of our experiences, we can co-create a culture that helps us sustain, motivate and support us all with compassion.

ADDITIONAL RESOURCES

Video resources and online information

You can get a sense of what it is like to attend a Round by watching an edited video of a Round on the Point of Care Foundation website. You can reach the following page by searching 'Schwartz Rounds' or 'Point of Care Foundation' on an internet search browser, going onto the Point of Care Foundation website and then clicking on 'Films' within the 'Evidence & Resources' link: www.pointofcarefoundation.org.uk/resource/watch-a-schwartz-round/

The Point of Care Foundation itself is full of useful information about Schwartz Rounds, and is a great place to look around, to find out more about Rounds and how they work. You can access this website by entering 'Schwartz Rounds' or 'Point of Care Foundation' into your internet search engine.

www.pointofcarefoundation.org.uk/our-programmes/schwartz-rounds/

FURTHER READING

Health and Care Professional Council. (HCPC, 2020) Reflecting on your practice and its emotional impact with Schwartz rounds. www.hcpc-uk.org/standards/meeting-our-standards/reflective-practice/types-of-reflective-practice/reflecting-on-your-practice-and-its-emotional-impact-with-schwartz-rounds/ [accessed June 2024]

Liverpool University and introducing Schwartz Rounds. www.youtube.com/watch?v=cw5LItLVmsA [accessed June 2024]

Newcastle Upon Tyne Schwartz Rounds. https://youtu.be/UJfwdrXW5tw?si=psmVBs_4uM689cT2 [Accessed June 2024]

NHS Providers. (2020). committees.parliament.uk/writtenevidence/10143/pdf/ [accessed June 2024)

Points of You See: https://points-of-you.com/ [accessed June 2024]

Robert, G., Philippou, J. and Leamy, M., et al. (2016). Exploring the adoption of Schwartz Center Rounds as an organisational innovation to improve staff well-being in England, 2009–2015. *BMJ Open, 7*, e014326. https://doi.org/10.1136/bmjopen-2016-014326 [accessed June 2024]

Schwartz, K. (1995). A Patient's Story. Boston: Boston Globe Magazine. A patient's story – The Boston Globe [accessed June 2024]

Smith, R. (2019) Schwartz rounds – A simple way to support staff and promote compassionate patient care. *BMJ Open.* https://blogs.bmj.com/bmj/2019/09/05/richard-smith-schwartz-rounds%e2%81%a0-a-simple-easily-implemented-way-to-support-staff-and-promote-compassionate-patient-care/ [accessed June 2024]

REFERENCES

Atkins, S., Pilnick, A., Maben, J. and Thompson, L. (2023) Storytelling and affiliation between healthcare staff in Schwartz Round interactions: A conversation analytic study. *Social Science & Medicine, 333*, 116–111.

Canzan, F., Saiani, L. and Mezzalira, E. et al. (2022) Why do nursing students leave bachelor program? Findings from a qualitative descriptive study. *BMC Nurs, 21*, 71. https://doi.org/10.1186/s12912-022-00851-z

Centre for the Advancement for Interprofessional Education (CAIPE). [accessed June 2024]

Clancy, D., Mitchell, A. and Smart, C. (2020). A qualitative exploration of the experiences of students attending interprofessional Schwartz Rounds in a University context. *Journal of Interprofessional Care, 34*(3), 287–296.

Driscoll, J. (2007) *Practising clinical supervision: A reflective approach for healthcare professionals*. 2nd edn. Edinburgh: Bailliere Tindall Elsevier.

Flanagan, E., Chadwick, R., Goodrich, J., Ford, C. and Wickens, R. (2019) Reflection for all healthcare staff: A national evaluation of Schwartz Rounds. *Journal of Interprofessional Care, 34*(1), 140–142. https://doi.org/10.1080/13561820.2019.1636008

Gibbs, G. (1998) *Learning by Doing: A Guide to Teaching and Learning Methods*. Oxford: Oxford Brooks University, Oxford.

Hamilton, D., Taylor, C. and Maben, J. (2023). How does a group reflection intervention (Schwartz rounds) work within healthcare undergraduate settings? *A realist review. Perspectives on medical education, 12*(1), 550.

Hill, J. E., Harris, C., Danielle L., C., Boland, P., Doherty, A. J., Benedetto, V., Gita, B. E. and Clegg, A. J. (2022) The prevalence of mental health conditions in healthcare workers during and after a pandemic: Systematic review and meta-analysis. *Journal of Advanced Nursing, 78*(6), 1551–1573. https://doi.org/10.1111/jan.15175

House of Commons Health and Social Care Committee. (2021) Workforce burnout and resilience in the NHS and social care

Irvine, D., Roger, S., Barrett, P., Obbard, K., Djwa, S., Risam, R., Zeffiro, A., Fong, D., Fitzpatrick, R., Betts, G. and Schmaltz, E. eds., (2023) *Future Horizons: Canadian Digital Humanities*. University of Ottawa Press.

Jones, L. and Green, J. (2006). Shifting discourses of professionalism: A case study of general practitioners in the United Kingdom. *Sociology of Health and Illness, 28*(7), 927–950. https://doi.org/10.1111/j.1467-9566.2006.00513.x

Maben, J., Taylor, C., Dawson, J., Leamy, M.C., McCarthy, I., Reynolds, E.F., Ross, S., Shuldham, C., Bennett, L. and Foot, C. (2018). A realist informed mixed-methods evaluation of Schwartz Center Rounds® in England.

Maben, J. and Taylor, C. (2021). Schwartz center rounds: An intervention to enhance staff well-being and promote organisational change. In *Connecting Healthcare Worker Well-Being, Patient Safety and Organisational Change: The Triple Challenge* (pp. 281–298). Cham: Springer International Publishing.

Maslach, C. and Leiter, M. P. (2016). Understanding the burnout experience: recent research and its implications for psychiatry. *World psychiatry, 15*(2), 103–111.

Morse, G., Salyers, M. P., Rollins, A. L., Monroe-DeVita, M. and Pfahler, C. (2012). Burnout in mental health services: A review of the problem and its remediation. *Administration and Policy in Mental Health and Mental Health Services Research, 39*(5), 341–352. https://doi.org/10.1007/s10488-011-0352-1

NHS Employers. (2024) Beating burnout in the NHS. Beating burnout in the NHS | NHS Employers [accessed June 2024].

NHS People Promise. (2024). www.england.nhs.uk/our-nhs-people/online-version/lfaop/our-nhs-people-promise/ [accessed June 2024]

Ng, L., Schache K. and Young M., et al. Value of Schwartz Rounds in promoting the emotional well-being of healthcare workers: A qualitative study. *BMJ Open, 13*, e064144. https://doi.org/10.1136/bmjopen-2022-064144

PoCF (2022). Schwartz Rounds in Higher Education Institutions Conference 2022. Available via https://www.pointofcarefoundation.org.uk/blog/schwartz-rounds-in-higher-educa tion-institutions-conference-2022/ last accessed 6/10/2025)

Point of Care Foundation. Schwartz Rounds. www.pointofcarefoundation.org.uk/our-programmes/staff-experience/schwartz-rounds-roles/ [accessed June 2024]

Point of Care Foundation. Schwartz Rounds. See: www.pointofcarefoundation.org.uk/our-programmes/staff-experience/about-schwartz-rounds/schwartz-rounds-in-higher-education/ [accessed June 2024]

Rider, E. A., Kurtz, S., Slade, D., Longmaid, H. E., Ho, M. J., Pun, J. K. H., Eggins, S. and Branch, W. T. (2014). The international charter for human values in healthcare: An interprofessional global collaboration to enhance values and communication in healthcare. *Patient Education and Counseling, 96*(3), 273–280. https://doi.org/10.1016/j.pec.2014.06.017

Russo-Netzer, P., Sinai, M. and Zeevi, M. (2020). Meaning in life and work among counsellors: A qualitative exploration. *British Journal of Guidance and Counselling, 48*(2), 209–226. https://doi.org/10.1080/03069885.2019.1625026

Simionato, G. K. and Simpson, S. (2018). Personal risk factors associated with burnout among psychotherapists: A systematic review of the literature. *Journal of Clinical Psychology, 74*(9), 1431–1456. https://doi.org/10.1002/jclp.22615

Winn, S. and Lindqvist S. (2019) Purposeful involvement of experts by experience. *The Clinical Teacher, 16*, 183–188. https://doi.org/10.1111/tct.13032

Wren, B. (2016). *True tales of organisational life*. London: Karnac.

Zervos, M. and Gishen, F. (2019). Reflecting on a career not yet lived: student Schwartz Rounds. *The Clinical Teacher, 16*(4), 409–411.

Zile, A., Owen, J., Orford, A. and Panagiotaki, G. (2024). Manuscript submitted for peer review.

Chapter 7
Gambling with health and well-being

Sally Hardy

INTRODUCTION

This chapter explores when inner challenges override healthy choices and behaviours. It addresses how self-help can be achieved, commencing with improving self-assessment of risky behaviours to become 'one's own nurse' (Hardy et al., 2019). Self-care enhances empathy as health professionals, and identifying and understanding entangled dynamics can help address early risks associated with long-term health and well-being. Recognizing when professional help is needed, the chapter offers evidence-based options for when friends, family, colleagues, or clients show risky gambling behaviours and addictive traits. Everyone gambles to some extent.

CASE STUDY

I work in the health care sector. I trained hard for my job, but my job has hit me hard. I have thought long and hard about where this all began. I guess I can blame my grandad. He used to religiously do the football pools and get me to run to the bookies with his bet. Most weekends we had small winnings that made Grandma laugh, and she'd ask for a new 'Sunday best' outfit. The losing weekends she would just hand us supper without a word. Family holidays beside the seaside, I was given lose change to play on the slot machines. Harmless fun, my parents called it.

At university most people wanted to go out drinking, partying, but I went back to my room playing video games, which, on a student loan, was my idea of saving money. I bought more equipment as the gaming got serious.

DOI: 10.4324/9781041057956-8

Eventually online gaming was for money. I won at first. I made over £600 winnings one night. This really got me buzzin'. I was enjoying myself.

My tutor noticed my grades were dropping. I let slip I had been gambling in a desperate attempt to get some sympathy. They gave me some links, like Gamblers Anonymous, and referred me to the well-being service. I read some of it, but the pull of the internet and all it offered was stronger. Months later, my parents got involved as I hadn't paid my rent, and they were really worried about me.

I took a year out and spent quite a bit of time working on my fitness. I started to feel better about myself and got myself a partner. I finally went back and completed my degree, and my partner and I moved in together. I really enjoyed working in emergency care and got into a good habit of work, homelife, and socializing.

Then we had our first baby. Sleep was a real issue. I delayed going home after work, ending up at the bookies looking at the horses, football, anything where I could earn some additional money. I thought this would make my partner happier and show I could provide for the baby. I started drinking and spending more time at the pub. I even asked Mum and Dad to lend me money – I said it was for a family holiday by the sea. I lost the lot in one binge session. I hated myself. Work noticed my lack of concentration, and I was put off work after an incident where I lost my rag.

My partner and child went to their parents, and I was given an ultimatum. I drank a bottle of whisky that night and took tablets. My partner rang back and, when I didn't pick up, phoned an ambulance. The ambulance crew were amazing. It made me realize what I had become. I reached out for help. I now have a sponsor, who appreciates gambling is a habit and needs to be managed. It's early days, but I really want to tackle this, and with the right help I think I can get my life back on track.

CRITICAL QUESTIONS

- What emotional and behavioural entangled dynamics, or patterns, can be identified from the case study?
- What role does pressure of work, money, and relationships have on some of the choices being made?

- When would an intervention be needed, if this person were a friend, relative, or colleague?
- When is a good time to seek professional help in this scenario?

GAMBLING WITH WELL-BEING

Work and life stressors are key risk factors that negatively affect mental and physical health, with enormous amounts of research that cannot be adequately covered in this chapter. Barnes et al. (2023) identified these as 'entangled themes', intertwined aspects of stressful working life that co-exist, making it difficult to prioritize which elements require intervention.

> *the entanglement of mental health problems, substance use, poor general health, and chronic pain . . . calls for implementation of a comprehensive health care integration approach, rather than management of these problems in isolation, or (risk) not identifying them at all.*
>
> (Barnes et al, 2023, p 10)

Pachi et al, (2023) identified a significant rise in anxiety and depression in those who remained 'frontline' carers during the Covid-19 pandemic. This was a traumatic episode for many with an increased risk of isolation, seeking solutions to work-related stress, increased alcohol and drug taking, and a lack of self-care, which can all lead to negative longer-term consequences.

Financial insecurity can affect a person's health-related behaviour. A global economic downturn in the UK, known as the 'Cost of Living Crisis', has many working people living in poverty, using food banks, and taking on additional work (Fitzpatrick et al, 2023; Munro et al, 2023). Escalating bills mean people gamble each month on whether to use their salary to feed the family or fill the fuel tank to get to and from school and work (McGloin, 2023).

It is well known that alcohol and drug addiction have negative consequences on health, with progressive and sometimes fatal health outcomes. Less is known about gambling behaviours, with many seeing this as a social problem. For nurses and other health professionals, their addictive behaviours are no greater or less than the general public, but many choose not to discuss or disclose their addiction for fear of losing their right to practice (Dunn, 2005).

WHEN GAMBLING BECOMES A PROBLEM

A changing pattern of gambling is related to availability via the internet (Sharman et al, 2019). Rogers et al. (2019) identified technology makes online gambling easier for people, with 51 per cent of individuals gambling via laptops, tablets, and mobile phones. These mobile devices offer easy access to gambling, with 97 per cent accessed from home and 13 per cent gambling online at work. Of the younger generation, (18- to 24-year-olds) 22 per cent gambled at work, 22 per cent while commuting, and 10 per cent in a social space, such as in a pub or club.

Gambling has negative connotations, like being seen as a cheat, or fraudster, someone of loose morals, weak-willed, unreliable, secretive, and dishonest, which may partly explain associations made between gambling and criminality (Jiang et al, 2023). Gamblers still experience stigma and a lack of compassion (National Research Council, 1999). Such negative representation has a strong impact on attitudes to gambling, although focus is placed most often on the individual, rather than placing emphasis of responsibility on the gaming industry itself.

Problem gambling is characterised by a compulsion to gamble and a preoccupation with gambling activity. Problem gambling often brings detriment to other social commitments, whether work, homelife, relationships, plus negative financial consequences. As gambling consequences start to spiral into family lives, there is associated harm, whether financial, emotional, and relational. Plus, there are physical and mental health implications. Gamblers are likely to have associated high alcohol intake, fueling poor choices while gambling, and a high association with other addictive behaviours, such as drug- and risk-taking (Thomas et al, 2008; McBride and Derevensky, 2012; McCarthy et al, 2023). In clinical settings, problem gambling is defined by the Diagnostic and Statistical Manual of Mental Disorders-5 (DSM-5) as a 'gambling disorder' which replaced the term 'pathological gambling' (American Psychiatric Association, 2000; 2013).

REFLECTIVE TASK 1

Read through the DSM-5 criteria below.

a. Persistent and recurrent problematic gambling behaviour leading to clinically significant impairment or distress, as indicated by the individual exhibiting four (or more) of the following in a 12-month period:
    1. Needs to gamble with increasing amounts of money to achieve the desired excitement.
    2. Is restless or irritable when attempting to cut down or stop gambling.

3. Has made repeated unsuccessful efforts to control, cut back, or stop gambling.
4. Is often preoccupied with gambling (e.g., having persistent thoughts of reliving past gambling experiences, handicapping or planning the next venture, thinking of ways to get money with which to gamble).
5. Often gambles when feeling distressed (e.g., helpless, guilty, anxious, depressed).
6. After losing money gambling, often returns another day to get even ('chasing' one's losses).
7. Lies to conceal the extent of involvement with gambling.
8. Has jeopardized or lost a significant relationship, job, or educational or career opportunity because of gambling.
9. Relies on others to provide money to relieve desperate financial situations caused by gambling.

b. The gambling behaviour is not better explained by a manic episode.

SPECIFY IF:

Episodic: Meeting diagnostic criteria at more than one time point, with symptoms subsiding between periods of gambling disorder for at least several months.
Persistent: Experiencing continuous symptoms, to meet diagnostic criteria for multiple years.

SPECIFY IF:

In early remission: After full criteria for gambling disorder were previously met, none of the criteria for gambling disorder have been met for at least 3 months but for less than 12 months.
In sustained remission: After full criteria for gambling disorder were previously met, none of the criteria for gambling disorder have been met during a period of 12 months or longer.

SPECIFY CURRENT SEVERITY:

Mild: 4–5 criteria met.
Moderate: 6–7 criteria met.
Severe: 8–9 criteria met.

(The Diagnostic and Statistical Manual of Mental Disorders,
5th Edition (section 312.31))

Reflective task 1: Now reflect on your own behaviour. What if you replaced the notion of gambling with either alcohol, eating, drug taking, or any other risky addiction adopted to deal with work and/or life's stressors?

GAMBLING TREATMENT OPTIONS

The National Health Service (NHS) long-term plan (2019) recognised the need to invest in specialist services to help more people with serious problem gambling, stating a need to understand the economic impact of gambling harm, plus getting the balance right between intervention, prevention, and treatments. Thomas, (2019) states that the scale of need does not currently match provision. Policy directives have moved from aiming for complete abstinence to a harm minimisation or 'safer' gambling approach to interventions and treatment options.

Most gambling treatment support occurs in dedicated specialist gambling service providers, which have diverse approaches. Evidence of long-term positive results is mixed and difficult to compare. Whether services should adopt theoretically or evidence-based treatments when there is only limited evidence from which to match best treatment options to individual's needs remains an issue (Petry, Ginley, and Rash, 2017; Tolchard et al, 2019).

Gamblers Anonymous (GA) is an international group who share their personal experiences of gambling in the hope of helping solve their common gambling problem experiences, working as a process of peer support. The individualised and private nature of a 12-step programme makes comparative evaluation problematic. The evidence there is for GA is that it can be as effective as any other active treatments (Marceaux et al., 2011; Stinchfield and Winters, 2001; Toneatto and Dragonetti, 2008). Schuler et al., (2016) undertook a review of GA and concluded there was limited evidence of effectiveness.

Although gambling treatment options have focused traditionally on adults, there is a growing problem with adolescent gambling, evidenced by the commissioning of the first gambling clinic for children and adolescents in the UK. Gambling-related treatment options frequently identified in the published literature are outlined in the comparative treatment table subsequently.

SELF-HELP STRATEGIES

Self-help has been shown to reduce the number of people with depression and anxiety from going into higher severity, particularly when used as an adjunct to other treatments. To date, self-help based on MI, CBT, and PNF has the best

Table 7.1 Gambling treatment options: a comparison of the evidence

Motivational interviewing (MI)	Cognitive behaviour therapy (CBT)	Personalised normative feedback (PNF)	Pharmaceutical options
MI is client centred and encourages commitment to change through personal decision making and planning (Rollnick and Miller, 1995). Systematic reviews of MI show effectiveness for conditions including 1. youth and adult drinking (Kohler and Hofmann, 2015; Vasilaki, Hosier, and Cox, 2006), 2. lifestyle issues (Rubak, Sandbæk, Lauritzen, and Christensen, 2005), and 3. health problems (Britt, Hudson, and Blampied, 2004).	CBT is adapted from Aaron Beck's (Beck, 2019) original cognitive therapy model for depression mixed with a range of behavioural treatments (e.g. exposure therapy primarily in the form of cue activation either in real-life situations or in imagination) with origins in Joseph Wolpe's systematic desensitisation (Wolpe and Reyna, 2013). Several cognitive and behavioural approaches have been described in the gambling literature as a useful treatment, including combining different aspects of cognitive-behaviour therapies through to third-wave integrative models of mindfulness-based CBT and all variants in between.	PNF is a person-centred approach commonly found in addictions treatment, which tailor's messages regarding their gambling behaviour using comparisons to others who gamble (Peter et al., 2019). PNF is often provided in a single session and reported in systematic reviews for alcohol-related issues across a range of subgroups (Dotson, Dunn, and Bowers, 2015; Pedersen, Parast, Marshall, Schell, and Neighbors, 2017).	The evidence for problem gambling using medication/pharmaceuticals alone is limited (Grant, Odlaug, and Schreiber, 2014; Pallesen et al., 2005, 2007). There is stronger evidence for having a combined approach, with psychological interventions (e.g., CBT) (Goslar, Leibetseder, Muench, Hofmann and Laireiter, 2018); however, the research evidence available is still small.

(Continued)

Table 7.1 (Continued)

Motivational interviewing (MI)	Cognitive behaviour therapy (CBT)	Personalised normative feedback (PNF)	Pharmaceutical options
Studies that show benefits indicate MI usefulness is in engaging participants to further enhance a self-help approach to problem gambling (Dimarco, Klein, Clark, and Wilson, 2009; Schilling, El-Bassel, Finch, Roman, and Hanson, 2002; Vella-Zarb, Mills, Westra, Carter, and Keating, 2015).	A summary of the published literature concludes such techniques have an initial effect in extinguishing gambling behaviour which was not maintained in follow-up (Barker and Miller, 1966, 1968; Goorney, 1968; Koller, 1972; Lester, 1980; McConaghy, Armstrong, Blaszczynski, and Allcock, 1983; McConaghy, Blaszczynski, Frankova et al, 1991; Seager, 1970)	Studies indicate superiority over no treatment, but less evidence when compared to any other active treatment. PNF is provided as a self-help format where the material was mailed out to gamblers or supplied over an internet programme (Cunningham et al., 2012, 2009; Hodgins et al., 2019, 2013, 2001). A primary meta-analysis finding was that PNF delivered alone without therapist input was more effective.	In a meta-analysis of 39 studies, Goslar et al. (2018) concludes that overall opioid antagonists and mood stabilisers produce a significant response in controlled studies, with most producing meaningful reductions in gambling severity and behaviours. However, there was no difference from placebo. This finding may be due to influential effects of a) being seen by someone, b) larger motivations to change and c) natural recovery over time.Goslar et al (2018) described the use of antidepressants (44 per cent), opioid antagonists (21 per cent), mood stabilisers (21 per cent), and a variety of other drugs (14 per cent). Medications as a single line of treatment have short-term benefits but limited evidence of long-term use. Opioid antagonists and mood stabilisers have the best evidence with other medications such as antidepressants being effective in combination with active psycho-social intervention.

Source: Hardy

evidence (refer to Table 7.1). Individual treatments are effective with gamblers at all stages of severity but are essential with those at the severest end. For many, the negative impact of problem gambling is what stimulates the need to undertake self-help solutions, including social interventions from family, employers, and other social networks, all of which have been identified as useful in limiting and reducing problem gambling activities (Kushnir et al, 2018).

Identifying inputs, outputs, and consequences based on work achieved to date, the gambling severity gauge approach collates information from all aspects of the individual gambler's personal situation and circumstances, and maps this to a systematic review of the evidence associated with treatment options (Hardy et al, 2019). Using this gambling severity gauge will allow a person (ideally working through the gauge with their family or friends or counsellor/practitioners) to identify a person's gambling state.

Start at the centre of the gauge. Then look left to right to identify a range of potential behaviours. Move up and out to identify associated treatment options. Working outward from the person at the centre, the first layer represents inputs and outputs of potential treatment options available, plus consequences of treatment modalities for that person, working along the spectrum of gambling activity. The gauge works by moving from left – low-level risk (0) – to right – high-level risk (5).

Higher levels 3–5 represents gambling at its most destructive and harmful, with significant suicide risk and self-destructive thoughts. Suicide prevention strategies are required as a matter of urgency.

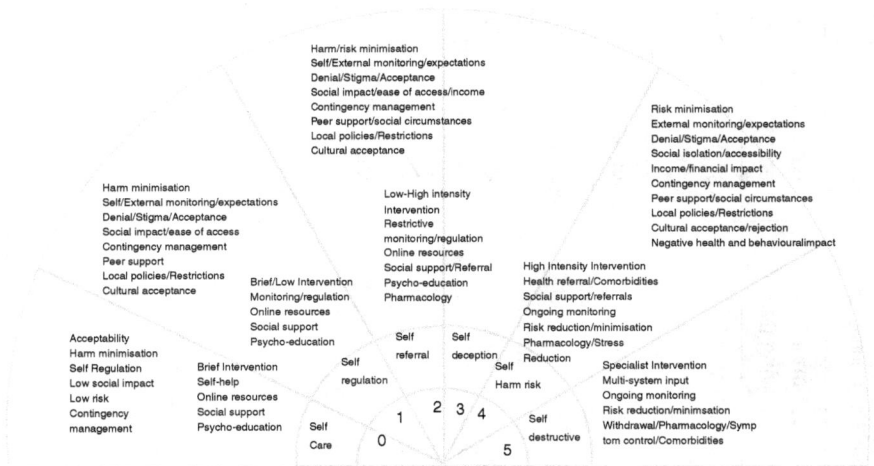

Figure 7.1 Person-centred gambling severity gauge (Hardy et al, 2019)

While self-help is useful, most people will need additional support to control their addiction successfully and sustain progress over time. Seeking input from those who have experienced problem gambling is considered an important element of helping gamblers learn strategies to reduce and even stop gambling behaviours. Couples therapy has been used successfully in some cases but remains untested with gamblers, perhaps through fear of exposure of revealing one's gambling state, plus going into therapy can place strain on the relationship of gambler and partner, so intra-partner communication through the therapist's facilitation style can affect each partner's contribution to changes placed on the relationship through therapy. In a qualitative critique of couple's therapy, Bertrand et al. (2008) concluded there is potential for this approach in gambling treatments, but to date little research has been achieved.

Reflection

Go through the gambling severity gauge. Replace the word 'gambling' with 'drinking', 'drug taking', 'eating', 'smoking' or any addictive behaviours that are or might be negatively affecting your health and well-being. Start at the centre of the gauge, then work left to right to identify a range of potential behaviours, and then move up and out to identify associated treatment options.

- What options of help are available, and which of the online self-help work-sheets (e.g., GamCare) might help you gain greater insight into gambling and/ or other addictive behaviours affecting your well-being?
- Identify who, (family, friends, or a trusted colleague) might do this reflective exercise with you, so that you can get their perspective on the level of severity compared to your own self-assessment. Complete this exercise.

WHEN DOES SELF-REGULATION NEED TO BECOME SELF-REFERRAL?

Shame and stigma can stop people from seeking help. The need for accessing the right support is essential in providing ourselves and our colleagues with a sensitive and personalised approach to achieving help. The Institute of Healthy Equality identified the following aspects where employers can provide essential support to their workforce. Recommendations include the following:

Embedding financial wellbeing and resilience into clinical pathways, consider-
ing how and where to co-locate services to support people. Provide workforce
training in how to identify at risk and support the workforce to contribute to
local approaches to address the rising cost of living, through considering the

whole person, when people present, and offer sign posting and support, ideally with minimal additional effort for the individual to help address the range of issues a person may need support with.

(Munro et al, 2023, p 6)

The evidence base for effective contingency management (CM) is vast, with the use of medication and beneficial effects as a combined approach to incentivised collaborative care. CM is an approach most frequently used with opioid addictions (DeFulio, 2023). The social feedback and support provided in the collaborative aspects of incentivisation is potentially the most highly effective aspect, as people build and rebuild trusting relationships with peers. With the advancement of digital technology, particularly for those who live far away from treatment facilities, the use of mobile devices has allowed remote connection, but should not be seen to fully replace face-to-face contact (Dallery et al, 2023).

LEARNING RESOURCES

Understanding a person's limitations and ability to manage risks is an important learning tool in all aspects of healthy behaviours.

1. Budgeting and financial management
    Look at some of the budgeting and debt management schemes readily available online, or through local citizens advice or other community groups and charities.
      Set a financial weekly or monthly limit to what is being spent on gambling, alcohol, cigarettes, chocolate, takeaways, etc.
      Agree to put some money aside each month to build up a reward fund to have available for a health-focused activity, (e.g., gym membership), or an agreed shared activity where others can enjoy time together (e.g., holidays, short breaks, trips out, cinema, bowling, shopping).
2. Balancing work-life commitments
    Make sure to use annual leave requirements, taking time away from work (which can become an addiction) and spending meaningful time with friends and family.
      Decide how much time to spend on yourself, and check how much time you give to helping or responding to others' requests for help.
3. Education – it's never too late
    The more you know, the better choices you can make, so educate yourself on matters that affect you and your health and well-being. It is never too late to

start to learn new ways of managing life stressors, and to change behaviours to help achieve long and healthy life. As seen in the case study, things change as your life and commitments change; so at each stage, be open to learning new strategies and ways of adapting to living well.

4. Toolkits and tips for behaviour change

There is an entire literature and a series of toolkits that can be accessed for understanding the science and practice of behaviour change. For example, the Easy, Attractive, Social and Timely (EAST) framework helps people set goals for change.

SUMMARY

Counselling and talking therapy help deal with and work to heal emotional wounds that are getting in the way of a person being able to choose and actively partake in a healthy lifestyle and associated life choices. The process of building trust and rapport with a therapist can help to identify specific personal vulnerabilities to relapse, help to expose any hidden triggers, and to devise a plan for the successful maintenance of sustained recovery.

Lessons learnt from exploring the evidence and effective options for investigating entangled dynamics of gambling with health and well-being raises the following issues.

- How often does regular monitoring and self-assessment (in terms of mental, physical, and financial health checks) against risks associated with nega- tively impacting our working lives, relationships, and longer-term career take place?
- Who are the people in trusting, collaborative relationships who can be relied upon to help address entangled themes and how to manage and prioritise these in seeking appropriate treatments in good time?
- How would you access what your employer offers to enable easy access to supportive, sensitive employer assistance services that enable all aspects aris- ing from work-related stressors to be managed and reported?

Some of the local initiatives experienced in the workplace to help address workplace stressors might include access to self-focused tools, such as mindfulness, journalling, and improving critical self-reflections, all of which will only be truly helpful and effective if organisations create a workplace well-being culture where these issues can be spoken about openly.

People spend so much time at work, and work closely with colleagues, so embracing these relationships as meaningful approaches for support, working collaboratively to enable each other's health and well-being as a natural or peer support approach, should be enhanced in the workplace and capitalised upon as part of our social contingency mechanisms. More examples are covered in more detail in other chapters in this book.

FURTHER READING

- Wyllie, C., Killick, E. and Kallman, A. (2023). *A review of gambling harm training materials for healthcare professionals*. tacklinggamblingstigma.com/wp-content/uploads/2023/04/A-Review-of-Gambling-Healthcare-Training-Tackling-Gambling-Stigma.pdf (accessed 21 February 2024)
- Real life gambling Stories from Gambling Watch UK
www.gamblingwatchuk.org/real-life-stories (accessed 21 February2024)
- The Counselling Directory. *10 of the most successful ways of overcoming gambling urges* www.counselling-directory.org.uk/counsellor-articles/the-10-most-successful-ways-of-overcoming-gambling-urges (accessed 21 February 2024)
- Gambling Anonymous (international) is a site with many resources aimed at helping and supporting people overcome their gambling behaviours.
www.gamblersanonymous.org/ga/content/20-questions (accessed 21 February 2024)
- GAMCARE: offers an online downloadable workbook to help identify aspects of gambling, plus monitoring its effect on different areas of life. It is free to download and offers a series of other activity worksheets that require an honest response to seeking help and gaining insight into gambling behaviours and associated emotional triggers, plus where and how to seek support. There are a series of worksheets included in the GamCare workbook, that are individually listed below, to make it easier to print off extra copies, and use these for yourself, family, or friend, or with clients.
www.gamcare.org.uk/self-help/self-help-resources/ (accessed 21 February 2024)
- The Mental Health Foundation website has a section on work-life balance and offers very practical tips for achieving a good work life balance, and many other useful resources addressing mental health.
www.mentalhealth.org.uk/explore-mental-health/a-z-topics/work-life-balance (accessed 21 February 2024)

REFERENCES

American Psychiatric Association. (2000) *Diagnostic Criteria from dsm-iv-tr*: American Psychiatric Pub

American Psychiatric Association. (2013) *Diagnostic and statistical manual of mental disorders (DSM-5®)*: American Psychiatric Pub

Barker, J. C. and Miller, M. (1966) Aversion therapy for compulsive gambling. *British Medical Journal*, *2*(5505), 115.

Barker, J. C. and Miller, M. (1968) Aversion therapy for compulsive gambling. *The Journal of Nervous and Mental Disease*, *146*(4), 285–302.

Barnes, A., Ye, G. Y., Ayers, C., Choflet, A., Lee, K. C., Zisook, S. and Davidson, J. E. (2023) Entangled: A mixed method analysis of nurses with mental health problems who die by suicide. *Nursing Inquiry*, *30*(2), e12537.

Beck, A. T. (2019) A 60-year evolution of cognitive theory and therapy. *Perspectives on Psychological Science*, *14*(1), 16–20.

Bertrand, K., Dufour, M., Wright, J. and Lasnier, B. (2008) Adapted couple therapy (ACT) for pathological gamblers: A promising avenue. *Journal of Gambling Studies, 24*(3), 393.

Britt, E., Hudson, S. M. and Blampied, N. M. (2004) Motivational interviewing in health settings: A review. *Patient Education and Counseling*, *53*(2), 147–155.

Cunningham, J. A., Hodgins, D. C., Toneatto, T. and Murphy, M. (2012) A randomized controlled trial of a personalized feedback intervention for problem gamblers. *PLoS One, 7*(2), e31586.

Cunningham, J. A, Hodgins, D. C., Toneatto, T., Rai, A. and Cordingley, J. (2009) Pilot study of a personalized feedback intervention for problem gamblers. *Behavior Therapy*, *40*(3), 219–224.

Dallery, J., Defulio, A. and Raiff, B. R. (2023) Digital contingency management in the treatment of substance use disorders. *Policy Insights from the Behavioral and Brain Sciences*, *10*(1), 51–58.

DeFulio, A. (2023) Dissemination of contingency management for the treatment of opioid use disorder. *Perspectives on Behaviour Science, 46*, 35–49.

Dimarco, I.D., Klein, D.A., Clark, V.L. and Wilson, G.T. (2009) The use of motivational interviewing techniques to enhance the efficacy of guided self-help behavioral weight loss treatment. *Eating Behaviors*, *10*(2), 134–136.

Dotson, K.B., Dunn, M.E. and Bowers, C.A. (2015) Stand-alone personalized normative feedback for college student drinkers: A meta-analytic review, 2004 to 2014. *PLoS ONE*, *10*(10), e0139518.

Dunn, D. (2005) Substance abuse among nurses – Defining the issue. *AORN Journal*, *82*(4), 572–596.

Fitzpatrick, S., Bramley, G., Treanor, M., Blenkinsopp, J., Johnsen, S. and McMordie, L. (2023) *Destitution in the UK 2023 [summary]*. Joseph Rowntree Foundation, York. www.jrf.org.uk/report/destitution-uk-2023 (last accessed 21/2/2024)

Goorney, A. (1968) Treatment of a compulsive horse race gambler by aversion therapy. *The British Journal of Psychiatry*, *114*(508), 329–333.

Goslar, M., Leibetseder, M., Muench, H.M., Hofmann, S.G. and Laireiter, A.R. (2018) Pharmacological treatments for disordered gambling: A meta-analysis. *Journal of Gambling Studies*, 1–31.

Grant, J.E., Odlaug, B.L., Black, D.W., Fong, T., Davtian, M., Chipkin, R. and Kim, S.W. (2014) A single-blind study of 'as-needed' ecopipam for gambling disorder. *Ann Clin Psychiatry*, *26*(3), 179–186.

Hardy, S., Chaplin, E., Tolchard, B., Flood, C. and Thomas, B. (2019) *A Systematic scoping Review of Treatment Outcomes and Delivery for Problem Gamblers*. Unpublished Report. LSBU

Hodgins, D.C., Cunningham, J.A., Murray, R. and Hagopian, S. (2019) Online self-directed interventions for gambling disorder: Randomized controlled trial. *Journal of Gambling Studies*, *35*(2), 635–651.

Hodgins, D.C., Currie, S.R. and el-Guebaly, N. (2001) Motivational enhancement and self help treatments for problem gambling. *Journal of Consulting and Clinical Psychology*, *69*(1), 50.

Hodgins, D.C., Fick, G.H., Murray, R. and Cunningham, J.A. (2013) Internet-based interventions for disordered gamblers: Study protocol for a randomized controlled trial of online self-directed cognitive-behavioural motivational therapy. *BMC Public Health*, *13*(1), 10–10.

Jiang, Y., Marcowski, P., Ryazanov, A. and Winkielman, P. (2023) People conform to social norms when gambling with lives or money. *Scientific Reports*, *13*(1), 853.

Kohler, S. and Hofmann, A. (2015) Can motivational interviewing in emergency care reduce alcohol consumption in young people? A systematic review and meta-analysis. *Alcohol and Alcoholism*, *50*(2), 107–117.

Koller, K.M. (1972) Treatment of poker-machine addicts by aversion therapy. *The Medical Journal of Australia*, *1*(15), 742.

Kushnir, V., Godinho, A., Hodgins, D.C., Hendershot, C.S. and Cunningham, J.A. (2018) Self-directed gambling changes: Trajectory of problem gambling severity in absence of treatment. *Journal of Gambling Studies*, 1–15.

Lester, D. (1980) The treatment of compulsive gambling. *International Journal of the Addictions*, *15*(2), 201–206.

Marceaux, J.C., Melville, C.L., Marceaux, J.C. and Melville, C.L. (2011) Twelve-step facilitated versus mapping-enhanced cognitive-behavioral therapy for pathological gambling: A controlled study. *Journal of Gambling Studies*, *27*(1), 171–190.

Mcbride, J., and Derevensky, J. (2012) Internet gambling and risk-taking among students: An exploratory study. *Journal of Behavioral Addictions*, *1*(2), 50–58.

McCarthy, S., Thomas, S.L., Pitt, H., Warner, E., Roderique-Davies, G., Rintoul, A. and John, B. (2023) "They loved gambling more than me." Women's experiences of gambling-related harm as an affected other. *Health Promotion Journal of Australia*, *34*(2), 284–293.

McConaghy, N., Armstrong, M., Blaszczynski, A. and Allcock, C. (1983) Controlled comparison of aversive therapy and imaginal desensitization in compulsive gambling. *The British Journal of Psychiatry*, *142*(4), 366–372.

McConaghy, N., Blaszczynski, A., Frankova, A., McConaghy, N., Blaszczynski, A. and Frankova, A. (1991) Comparison of imaginal desensitisation with other behavioural treatments of pathological gambling. A two- to nine-year follow-up. *British Journal of Psychiatry*, *159*(3), 390–393.

McGloin, S. (2023) Cost-of-living crisis impacts the nursing and midwifery professions. *Occupational Medicine*, *73*(7), 385–387.

Munro, A., Allen, J. and Marmot, M. (2023) *The rising cost of living: A review of interventions to reduce impacts on health inequalities in London*. London: Institute of Health Equity. www.instituteofhealthequity.org/resources-reports/evidence-review-cost-of-living-and-health-inequalities-in-london/click-here-to-read-the-report.pdf (last accessed 21/2/2024)

National Health Service. (2019) *The NHS long term plan*. www.longtermplan.nhs.uk/ (last accessed 21/2/2024)

National Research Council. (1999) Committee on the social and economic impact of pathological gambling: A critical review. *Gambling Concepts and Nomenclature*, *2*.

Pachi, A., Kavourgia, E., Bratis, D., Fytsilis, K., Papageorgiou, S.M., Lekka, D., Sikaras, C. and Tselebis, A., (2023) Anger and aggression in relation to psychological resilience and alcohol abuse among health professionals during the first pandemic wave. *Healthcare*, *11*(14), 2031.

Pallesen, S., Mitsem, M., Kvale, G., Johnsen, B. and Molde, H. (2005) Outcome of psychological treatments of pathological gambling: A review and meta-analysis. *Addiction*, *100*(10), 1412–1422.

Pallesen, S., Molde, H., Arnestad, H.M., Laberg, J.C., Skutle, A., Iversen, E., Støylen, I.J., Kvale, G. and Holsten, F. (2007) Outcome of pharmacological treatments of pathological gambling: A review and meta-analysis. *Journal of Clinical Psychopharmacology*, *27*(4), 357–364.

Pedersen, E.R., Parast, L., Marshall, G.N., Schell, T.L. and Neighbors, C. (2017) A randomized controlled trial of a web-based, personalized normative feedback alcohol intervention for young-adult veterans. *Journal of Consulting and Clinical Psychology*, *85*(5), 459.

Peter, S.C., Brett, E.I., Suda, M.T., Leavens, E.L., Miller, M.B., Leffingwell, T.R. and Meyers, A.W. (2019) A meta-analysis of brief personalized feedback interventions for problematic gambling. *Journal of Gambling Studies*, 1–18.

Petry, N.M., Ginley, M.K. and Rash, C.J. (2017) A systematic review of treatments for problem gambling. *Psychology of Addictive Behaviors*, *31*(8), 951–961.

Rogers, R., Wardle, H., Sharp, C., Wood, S., Hughes, K., Davies, T., Dymond, S. and Bellis, M. (2019). *Gambling as a Public Health Issue in Wales*. Bangor University.

Rollnick, S. and Miller, W.R. (1995) What is motivational interviewing? *Behavioural and Cognitive Psychotherapy*, *23*(4), 325–334.

Rubak, S., Sandbæk, A., Lauritzen, T. and Christensen, B. (2005) Motivational interviewing: A systematic review and meta-analysis. *British Journal General Practice*, *55*(513), 305–312.

Seager, C. (1970) Treatment of compulsive gamblers by electrical aversion. *The British Journal of Psychiatry*, *117*(540), 545–553.

Schilling, R.F., El-Bassel, N., Finch, J.B., Roman, R.J. and Hanson, M. (2002) Motivational interviewing to encourage self-help participation following alcohol detoxification. *Research on Social Work Practice*, *12*(6), 711–730.

Schuler, A., Ferentzy, P., Turner, N.E., Skinner, W., McIsaac, K.E., Ziegler, C.P. and Matheson, F.I. (2016) Gamblers Anonymous as a recovery pathway: A scoping review. *Journal Of Gambling Studies*, *32*(4), 1261–1278.

Sharman, S., Murphy, R., Turner, J.J. and Roberts, A. (2019) Trends and patterns in UK treatment seeking gamblers: 2000–2015. *Addictive Behaviors*, *89*, 51–56.

Stinchfield, R. and Winters, K.C. (2001) Outcome of Minnesota's gambling treatment programs. *Journal of Gambling Studies*, *17*(3), 217–245. https://doi.org/10.1023/A:1012268322509

Thomas, R. (2019) The Bedpan: The NHS must take gambling seriously. *Health Service Journal*. 20 May 2019

Thomas, S.A., Piterman, L., and Jackson, A.C. (2008) Problem gambling: What do general practitioners need to know and do about it? *Medical Journal of Australia*, *189*(3), 135.

Tolchard, B., Hardy, S., Chaplin, E. and Flood, F. (2019) A systematic review of effective treatment for gambling problems. Unpublished Report LSBU.

Toneatto, T., and Dragonetti, R. (2008) Effectiveness of community-based treatment for problem gambling: A quasi-experimental evaluation of cognitive-behavioral vs. twelve-step therapy. *American Journal on Addictions*, *17*(4), 298–303.

Vasilaki, E.I., Hosier, S.G. and Cox, W.M. (2006) The efficacy of motivational interviewing as a brief intervention for excessive drinking: A meta-analytic review. *Alcohol and Alcoholism*, *41*(3), 328–335.

Vella-Zarb, R.A., Mills, J.S., Westra, H.A., Carter, J.C. and Keating, L. (2015) A Randomized controlled trial of motivational interviewing + self-help versus psychoeducation + self-help for binge eating. *International Journal of Eating Disorders*, *48*(3), 328–332.

Wolpe, J. and Reyna, L.J. (2013) *Behavior therapy in psychiatric practice: The use of behavioral procedures by psychiatrists*. Elsevier.

Chapter 8

In search of meaning through making

Jonathan Webster and Holly Sandiford

INTRODUCTION

Throughout this chapter, we plan to explore the importance of creative arts in maintaining well-being. We draw from personal experience by presenting our stories through the use of vignettes. Upon reflection of our personal journeys, we search for our own creative influences, which in turn have impacted our learning 'through making'. We consider reflections as you would when looking into a kaleidoscope and seeing many colours and forms within the context of application to the 'real world' context and what has shaped and influenced our own creative and professional practice. Our reflections and critical thinking will help develop a greater understanding of the process of 'meaning through making', through the lens of our own work. By the end of the chapter, we hope you will have an enriched understanding for your own self, from which to explore opportunities for creative learning, wider contextual understanding and personal application.

MEANING THROUGH MAKING AND CREATIVITY

The use and recognition of the importance of the creative arts is not new in supporting personal well-being. Interest has grown over the past decades, influenced by economics and psychology, with 'contributions' from the development studies and sociology (McLellan et al, 2012). Engaging with the creative arts as a 'tool' for both 'therapeutic value' and 'quality of life' is gaining increasing recognition (Cohen, 2006) in which therapeutic impact has been demonstrated for people living with trauma (Gutheil and Heyman, 2016). In addition, there has been an increased understanding of the importance of creative arts to support personal growth (Reynolds, 2010) throughout our life span (Gutheil and Heyman, 2016).

DOI: 10.4324/9781041057956-9

Creativity can take many forms, including visual art, singing, reciting literature, drama, dance and movement. Basford (2022) states that we are all born creative, sometimes we just lose that little part of ourselves. Noise et al. (1999) identified in their study the positive impact of theatrical training on the cognitive skills of older adults. Zarobe and Bungay (2017) reported a positive impact of creative activities on the well-being and health of children and young people, validating findings from Bungay and Vella Burrows, (2013) as the following:

- Increased self-esteem
- Sense of achievement
- Empowerment
- Social skills
- Promotion of social engagement

The positive impact of music as a therapeutic intervention for older people's physical and mental health, while living in nursing homes is also reported, in which music 'enhances well-being for the body and soul' (Wijk et al. 2021; 1).

From a professional health and care perspective, it is recognised that creativity can enable greater emotional intelligence which itself provides an opportunity to learn more about oneself, leading to greater professional effectiveness and compassion shown in care delivery, which cascades into the nurturing of creative workplace cultures (Coats, 2006). This highlights how creativity can lead to greater self-awareness, which in turn can positively impact the settings (contexts) in which we work.

Integral to being outwardly creative is the importance of being inwardly creative, recognising the positive impact on personal well-being of creativity that starts with the 'person' that nourishes the mind, body and soul as a journey of development and growth. In practice, this means that focussing on 'self' and personal creativity can act as the starting point of a journey in which creativity is awakened. In a world that is increasingly busy and pressurised with a focus on 'doing', reconnecting with one's own senses can be seen as being intrinsically important, linking to well-being drawing on the five senses of sight, hearing, smell, taste and touch.

In the two vignettes that follow, the place of nature, creativity and well-being are intrinsically linked. We explore how spending time in nature, through active engagement, demonstrates the positive impact on well-being (Richardson et al, 2021) through experiencing nature and the world around us by drawing on our senses in which we blend mind and body through activity (action).

VIGNETTE 1: JONATHAN CONNECTING WITH CLAY

Journey of Reflection and Creativity through working with Clay
(by Jonathan Webster)
Spiral of movement,
Silence, thought, quiet,
Senses take over,
Silence, thought, quiet,
Hands and mind in coordinated concentration,
Silence, thought, quiet,
New life, new form, new shape,
Silence, thought, quiet,
Reawakening of creativity,
Silence, reflection, quiet.

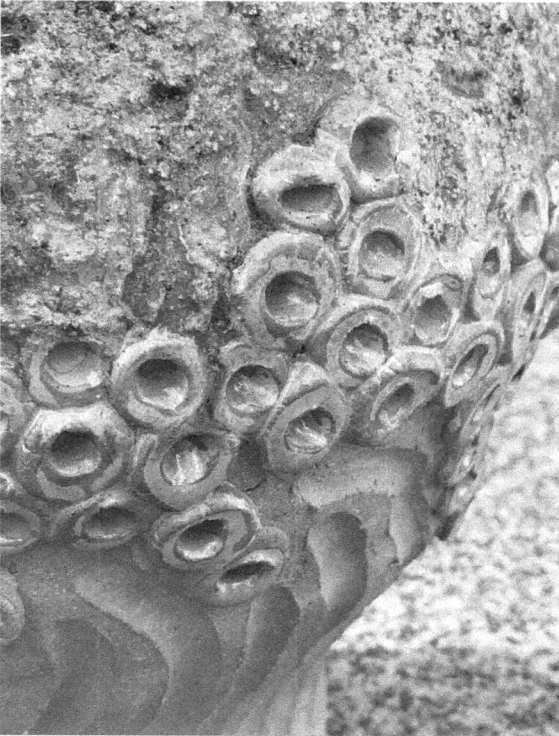

Figure 8.1 'Rock Pool Sculpture' 2020, partial glazed ceramic by Jonathan Webster

My reawakening to working with clay occurred after a 30-year time lapse. Life became busy and commitments took over. Some might describe this as the 'business of life' both at work and home. Long days at work became all-consuming. I know now that I looked down, focussing on 'getting through'. I did the best I could, and then suddenly 'it' stopped. I was made redundant after 30+ years, and my working world came to a screeching halt.

Reacquainting myself with clay became a focal point of activity. Skills learnt long ago that had once been a central focus in my teenage years started to re-emerge. I became inquisitive as to a life from a deeply buried earlier chapter. Attending weekly day time classes, I lost myself in working with clay. The hours spent each week at class was 'my time'. I lost myself in my creative work – wedging clay, creating, experimenting and decorating. I connected the physical activity of doing with thinking, which released the creativity that had become locked away over time. My mind and body became one. I sensed a feeling of release and well-being that I almost became addicted to. I so looked forward to my weekly classes. I could be 'just' me!

My brain was able to 'settle'. I felt a calmness, and I lost myself in the act of working with clay. I experienced a sense of respect between the creator (me) and the clay I was working with, in a creative symbiotic relationship that had been lost over time.

Some weeks I chatted to people, other weeks I was happy to work in purposeful silence in which my spirit, mind and body was in control. My senses took over. I imagined and saw nature – the greenness of Spring, the sleep of Winter, waves crashing against the shore, the smell and taste of salt in the air and the earthiness of the clay forming in my hands.

Over time I have recognised the centrality of the relationship between the potter and clay. Clay in its raw state isn't an inanimate object. I have to work with the clay; I need to recognise its potential and also its limitations. I need to 'listen' to the clay with my hands. Sensing what form and direction it is taking me in. How do I need to form a connectivity to support what I want to achieve?

Centering a piece of clay on a potter's wheel requires skill. Not only in the technique used but in the relationship and connectivity between the clay and me (the potter). My mind connects to my hands, and my hands connect to my mind, in which both connect with the clay. I concentrate and lose myself, thinking in the movement and feeling the form that starts to emerge which is a creation between the clay and me.

A sense of calm descends over me, and I focus on the rhythmic movement of the clay on the wheel. An activity that connects me back over thousands of years to the early potters working with raw materials and with the origins of clay in the natural world.

I am able to work at a pace that reflects my needs at the time and what the clay is prepared to give. I've learnt lifting a pot can't be rushed. As rushing usually leads to 'disaster'! Instead, I concentrate and focus on what I am doing. I breathe evenly. I stay calm and in control, and work with the clay, bringing mind and hands together. If I listen to the clay through my hands, the clay tells me if I am rushing and if I need to slow down, which I then do. A harmonious connection and creative expression.

REFLECTIONS ON VIGNETTE 1

This vignette captured a period of time and journey for the author. It describes a gradual re-emergence of practical skills and an intuitive knowing, an understanding through using clay to connect mind, body and soul, as a sense of emergent connectedness, a natural well-being. Through greater insight and creative learning there is a synergy in which there is an opportunity to 'externalise' and give meaning to inner thoughts and feelings, from which to express what is 'out there', alongside what was 'hidden', not being expressed (Coulson and Stickley, 2002).

In referring to art-based research, Coulson and Stickley (2002:87) state:

> Artistic expression appeals to the inner person and allows creative narrative of the individual's inner world.

There is also an embedded resonance with the view of Freshwater (2004), who identified that through creativity, greater emotional intelligence can occur, which provides an opportunity to learn both about oneself and the way in which one relates with others. Social connection with others provides opportunity for shared learning, which promotes a sense of social inclusivity and a patchwork of lived experiences (Hughes et al., 2021) within the group. Working with clay, as described by Jonathan, provides an opportunity to acknowledge the 'inner' person. However, facilitated through creative learning, the ability to start looking upwards and outwards to see and connect with the surrounding world is embraced. To see a natural world that is beyond the immediate limited context at that time provides insight into a world that has endless future opportunities and innate connections.

Learning through creating doesn't stay purely within a focus of personal, self-focused creativity. Learning about self can translate to the practice setting as it enables an ability to look upward and outwards, posing the questions 'how does the creative me relate and translate to the professional me?' and 'how does this creative awareness positively impact on my own physical and psychological well-being?'

As a registered nurse, the centrality of person-centredness has become increasingly important in my own (Jonathan's) practice. My creative interconnectedness, as spirals of learning, has enabled a closer connection and authentic valuing of the 'person'. Connecting mind, body and soul through being creative and embracing embedded learning can enable new ways of working, knowing and learning (if nurtured and enabled to flourish) that translates and becomes a cultural norm that enhances potential for human interaction and connectedness within the practice setting.

VIGNETTE 2: HOLLY'S WORKING WITH NATURE

My creative practice is focused on deepening my connection with the natural world and encouraging others to do the same. Going and being outside reconnects me with myself, reminding me I am part of nature, not separate from it. The more time I spend surrounded by nature, the more conscious I become of my responsibility to take more care of it. Nature awakens a sense of aliveness within me, reminding me of what it means to be human. It is essential for the maintenance of my well-being.

As I delve into creative exploration and embrace new ideas, I sense a gentle awakening in the centre of my chest. This feeling serves as my compass, guiding my creative decisions. If something does not give me this feeling, then I will try something else.

My photography involves analogue techniques and camera-less methods. Relying on old-fashioned cameras and creating images without using a physical camera. Before I create any artwork, I spend time in the location I am working with, whether that is the woods, a broad/water or a meadow. This allows me to tune into my surroundings and align my senses. If I still feel blocked creatively, then I experiment with exercises, such as drawing, sound recording or taking tree rubbings. The outside natural world becomes my studio.

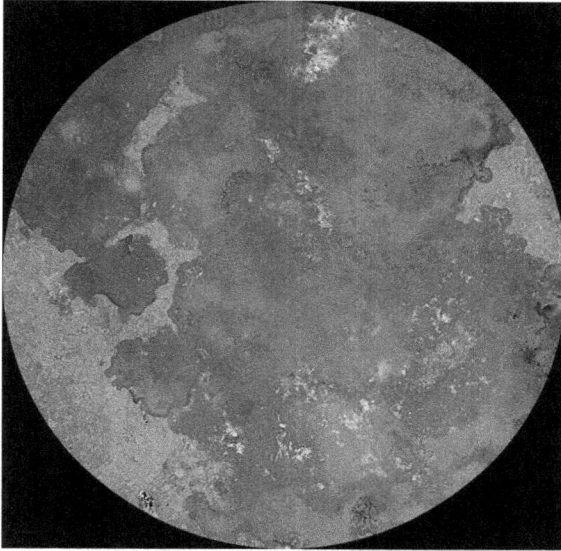

Figure 8.2 *Space and Soil* (2023). Soil painted onto expired photographic paper by Holly Sandiford

I co-create my work with nature and enjoy that I am not the only one in control of the artwork. I had a realisation that what I find in nature is so perfect and beautiful that I would prefer to work with it rather than trying to emulate it. This often entails working directly with plants and soil. For example, using soil to paint on expired photographic paper. The different PH levels and chemicals in the soils then interact differently with the paper, creating a variety of colours and patterns. Another example includes using an old camera to take photographs of the canopy of trees and then boiling the film roll in twigs, lichen, blossom and leaves that have fallen from that same tree! It creates a beautiful, dreamy effect with unexpected colours in the developed photographs.

Chance plays a big role in my work process, and I often produce unsuccessful outcomes. Being at ease with failure is an essential part of my creative practice. A lot of my photographs do not turn out well, but the excitement when they do is indescribable. Working in this way helps me tap into my playful, childlike side that often feels overshadowed by the demands and constraints of the modern world. I have a lot of responsibility in my life in my role as director of ArtatWork, a creative health not-for-profit, caring responsibilities and being a single mum to three girls. For me, being creative is essential to my well-being. Without it the world just feels somehow less.

It is also important for me that my work is accessible to everyone. This is definitely influenced by working with people with such different needs and coming from a lower socio-economic background. To reach beyond galleries, such as in mental health settings (e.g. a recent commission for hospital rooms), so that it can also help others see the world in a different light.

By being in nature and prioritising self-care, I allow my creativity to flourish. My creative practice not only nurtures my spirit but also enables me to inspire and support others effectively in their well-being journey.

REFLECTIONS LINKED TO VIGNETTE 2

This vignette emphasises the connection between creative practice and the natural world for the author. It highlights that deepening our connection to, and immersing ourselves in, nature, especially through creative activities, can enhance well-being. The author's practice supports current research, which shows that participating in creative activities can improve mental health by promoting feelings of autonomy and empowerment (National Centre for Creative Health, 2021). It is also important to the author that the work she creates benefits others. By inspiring them and encouraging them to see the world differently and the joy that can come from that. Recent studies, such as those published by Max-Planck-Gesellschaft (2023), confirm that even just viewing art can enhance mood and well-being.

The importance of self-care through creativity is clear in the author's narrative. Creative practices both promote personal and communal well-being, building a stronger bond with both oneself and nature. Combining this with a deep connection with nature, the creative process has the potential to bring balance and meaning to life, thus helping to manage the challenging demands of everyday life and the workplace.

The author uses creativity and nature to inspire others in community-based arts for well-being workshops. Participating in play and creation, with no expectations or judgements, can have a profound impact on well-being, especially when this experience is shared with others. Viewing the world through a creative lens can help more difficult thoughts and more negative ways of perceiving the world to subside. This collective engagement can be especially therapeutic for those who find constant social pressure exhausting, because they can engage when they like or stay silent and just enjoy making.

Delivering creative sessions in a natural environment or bringing nature indoors, if this is not possible, amplifies this positive effect on well-being. Research by Richardson et al. (2021) emphasises that spending time in nature can significantly enhance mental well-being. The concept of 'moments, not minutes' suggests that even brief moments of connection with nature can have a profound impact on reducing stress and improving overall well-being. Nature connection is more predictive of a sense of life being worthwhile than socio-economic status.

CREATIVE ACTIVITIES

We have discussed how combining creativity and nature can significantly enhance well-being by helping individuals relax, feel grounded and reconnect with their authentic selves. Here are some simple arts and nature ideas that you can try at home to boost your mental and emotional well-being.

Texture touch and draw

- **Activity:** While walking, touch different natural textures like tree bark, leaves or stones. Use a small sketchbook and a pencil to make quick rubbings or drawings of the textures you feel.
- **Materials:** Small sketchbook, pencil or crayon.

NATURE MANDALA

- **Activity:** Collect natural items such as leaves, flowers and stones during the walk. Arrange them into a mandala on the ground.
- **Materials:** Natural items collected during the walk.

MINDFUL LISTENING:

- **Activity:** Find a quiet spot to sit and close your eyes. Listen to the sounds of nature for a few minutes. Afterwards, draw or write about what you heard.
- **Materials:** Small notebook and pen.

BLIND CONTOUR DRAWING:

- **Activity:** Choose an object in nature, like a tree or flower, and draw it without looking at your paper. This helps enhance observation skills and creativity.
- **Materials:** Small sketchbook, pencil.

COLLECT AND COLLAGE:

- **Activity:** Collect small flat items like leaves, petals and feathers. Use them to create a collage in your sketchbook.
- **Materials:** Small sketchbook, glue stick, collected items.

DIRECTIONAL DECISION WITH WOODEN SPOON:

- **Activity:** Use a wooden spoon to decide which direction to walk. Throw the spoon and follow the direction it points to explore new paths.
- **Materials:** Wooden spoon.

SHAPE WALK:

- **Activity:** Focus on finding natural objects that match a specific shape, like circles or triangles. Sketch or photograph these objects.
- **Materials:** Small sketchbook and pencil, or mobile phone camera.

REFLECTIVE QUESTIONS

- Within my life, how do I experience and seek out opportunities for creativity? When I do, how does it make me feel?
- What insights have I gained reading Vignettes 1 and 2?
- Within my work context, what opportunities do I have to explore learning with others through creativity?
- What steps do I need to take to explore creativity further both for myself and others I work with?

SUMMARY

In this chapter, we drew on our personal experiences to explore how engaging with the arts, especially when combined with nature, can improve both personal and community well-being and in creating a better work/life balance. We showed that creativity in any form, whether through clay or alternative photography, helps us to reconnect with ourselves and the world that we experience daily.

Through the sharing of our personal vignettes, we highlighted how returning to creative practices, like Jonathan's work with clay, can reignite a sense of purpose and peace. Similarly, Holly's deep connection with nature through her socially engaged arts practice has the potential to promote both belonging and well-being. They also reveal that creativity, as well as being enjoyable in itself, can build community, improve resilience to challenging work situations and deepen our connection to ourselves, the natural world and to other people.

As you think about what we have discussed, consider how these ideas might inspire your own creative journey. This could be through going to a gallery to look at art, spending time in nature, observing something new in your daily routine, trying our simple activities or finding small moments to create in the way you like the best. It is not about creating a perfect piece of art or craft; it is about taking time for yourself and enjoying the process.

Everyone can be creative, and in a fast-paced world, the simple act of 'making' – whether with clay, a camera or your hands – reminds us of who we truly are as human beings.

FURTHER READING

Braiding Sweetgrass: Indigenous Wisdom, Scientific Knowledge, and the Teachings of Plants" by Robin Wall Kimmerer (2013)

Gadsby, F (2023) By My Hands, A Potters Apprenticeship, Penguin, Dublin: Ireland

The Nature Fix: Why Nature Makes Us Happier, Healthier, and More Creative" by Florence Williams (2017)

Your Brain on Art: How the Arts Transform Us" by Susan Magsamen and Ivy Ross (2023)

The Language of Trees: A Rewilding of Literature and Landscape" by Katie Holten (2023)

Entangled Life: How Fungi Make Our Worlds, Change Our Minds & Shape Our Futures" by Merlin Sheldrake (2020)

The power of pottery – rebuilding confidence through creativity, www.southwestlondonics.org.uk/local-stories/the-power-of-pottery-rebuilding-confidence-through-creativity/

WEBSITES/SOCIAL MEDIA PLATFORMS

64 Million Artists: This organisation promotes creativity and Well-being through challenges, workshops, and community engagement, encouraging everyone to tap into their creative potential. **Website: 64millionartists. com. Twitter/X: @64M_Artists**

National Centre for Creative Health (NCCH): Focuses on the role of creativity in health and Well-being, providing research, resources, and forums for discussion. **Twitter/X: @NCCH_UK. Website: ncch.org.uk**

Creative Health: The Arts for Health and Well-being (All-Party Parliamentary Group on Arts, Health and Well-being): A comprehensive report providing data, case studies, and policy recommendations on the use of the arts in health and social care settings. **Website: artshealthandWell-being.org.uk**

Arts and Health South West (AHSW): Promotes and supports the arts in health, offering a wealth of resources, research reports, and case studies. **Website: ahsw.org.uk**

REFERENCES

Basford, J. (2022) Forgive yourself for railed resolutions and focus on achievable change instead. February 2, 2022. *The P&J*. Available via www.pressandjournal.co.uk/fp/opinion/3909186/johanna-basford-forgive-failed-resolutions-focus-achievable-changes-opinion/ (last accessed 22 Oct 2024)

Bungay, H. and Vella Burrows, T. (2013) The effects of participating in creative activities in the health and wellbeing of children and young people: A rapid review of the literature. *Perspectives in Public Health*, 131, pp 45–52

Coats, E. (2006) *Opening Doors on Creativity: Resources to Awaken Creative Working*. Royal College of Nursing Institute. London: England

Cohen, G. (2006) Research on creativity and ageing: The positive impact of the arts on health and illness. *Generations*, 30 (1), pp 7–15

Coulson, P., Stickley, T. (2002) Finding a voice – Artistic expression and practice development, *Practice Development in Health Care*, 1 (2), pp 85–97

Freshwater, D. (2004) Emotional intelligence: Developing emotional literate training in mental health. *Mental Health Practice*, 8 (4), pp 12–15

Gutheil, I. and Heyman J. (2016) Older adults and creative arts: Personal and interpersonal change. *Activities, Adaptation & Aging*. 40, pp 169–179. https://doi.org/10.1080/01924788.2016.1194030

Hughes, M., Whitaker, L. and Rugendyke, B. (2021) 'Yesterday i couldn't see. tomorrow's sun shines now': Sharing migrant stories through creative arts to foster community connections and wellbeing. *Journal of Intercultural Studies*, 42 (5), pp 541–560 https://doi.org/10.1080/07256868.2021.1971170

Max-Planck-Gesellschaft. (2023) "Viewing art can improve our mood and well-being." *ScienceDaily*. 5 May 2023. <www.sciencedaily.com/releases/2023/05/230505101654.htm>.

McLellan, R., Galton M., Steward S. and Page, C. (2012) *The impact of creative initiatives on wellbeing: A literature review*. Creativity Culture and Education Newcastle upon Tyne: England

National Centre for Creative Health. (2021). *Creative Health Review*. Retrieved from https://ncch.org.uk/creative-health-review

Noise, H., Noiice, T., Perrig-Chiello, P. and Perrig, W. (1999) Improving memory in older adults by instructing them in professional actors' learning strategies. *Applied Cognitive Psychology*, 13, pp 315–328. https://doi.org/10.1002/(SICI)1099-0720 (199908)

Reynolds, F. (2010). 'Colour and communion': Exploring the influences of visual art-making as a leisure activity on older women's subjective well-being. *Journal of aging studies*, 24 (2), pp. 135–143.

Richardson, M., Passmore, H-A., Lumber, R., Thomas, R. and Hunt A. (2021) Moments, not minutes: The nature-wellbeing relationship. *International Journal of Wellbeing*, 11 (1), pp 8–33. https://doi.org/10.5502/ijw.v11i1.1267

Wijik, H., Neziraj, M. and Nilsson, A, et al (2021) Exploring the use of music as an intervention for older people living in nursing homes. *Nursing Older People*, https://doi.org/10.7748/nop.2021.e1361

Zarobe, L. and Bungay, H. (2017) The role of arts activities in developing resilience and mental wellbeing in children and young people a rapid review of the literature. *Perspectives in Public Health*, 137 (6), pp 337–347. https://doi.org/10.1177/1757917712283

Chapter 9

Staying in the game
Effective strategies for achieving long-term career goals

Rebekah Hill, Julia Hubbard and Lorna Sankey

INTRODUCTION

Working in health and social care is demanding both mentally and physically, with work patterns often taking a social and emotional toll on the individual. It can be hard to stay in the game, to keep working in a care environment when there are so many continued challenges to negotiate.

The reasons for staff leaving health and social care roles are varied and complex. It is possible to identify some common themes, but deciding to leave a healthcare career is usually due to an interplay of multiple factors (Ball et al., 2022; Pressley & Garside, 2023). Things that cause staff to leave can be referred to as 'push' factors, whilst things that keep staff working in healthcare are called 'pull' factors (Glogowska et al., 2007). It is important to consider both perspectives – factors that cause staff to leave as well as exploring how and why they stay when considering effective workforce retainment and retention strategies.

This chapter will consider the challenges and solutions to staying in the game, as a process of retaining qualified healthcare professionals in health and social care careers, as highly effective compassionate and caring members of the workforce. We explore first the background to difficulties surrounding staff retention in healthcare, before moving to consider organisational strategies that have been found to be most effective. Woven throughout is a discussion about well-being factors, and a series of reflective tasks to consider, from an individual perspective to help enable you and your colleagues (as any other registered healthcare professionals) to remain inspired to continue working in the health and care professions you chose.

DOI: 10.4324/9781041057956-10

CASE STUDY 1

ELISE, A NEWLY REGISTERED NURSE, ASKS – WHERE DO I BELONG?

I used to look forward to coming to work. I am not sure if I can pinpoint when I started feeling sick and panicky before a shift, as it just crept up on me. I really enjoyed my undergraduate programme. The mix of theory and practice. Plus, we'd have time in 'uni' on study days and then there would be specific time on the wards, on clinical days. I loved being super nummary when on the wards, which meant I wasn't counted in the staffing numbers on the placements I attended – which meant I had more flexibility and freedom. I had the chance to maximise my learning opportunities because I had the freedom to have more choice over what I did. I could watch novel investigations and procedures, decline some things I didn't want to do, but also, I could be part of a team on a ward or department.

I used to move wards every few weeks and loved learning about all the different specialties and working in the various teams. Although all this excitement of doing new things was great, I began to get tired of the constant moving around, feeling like a vagrant, not knowing where I belonged. By the time I was in my third year, I felt I just wanted to stay in one place. I yearned to get to know the job better and be really understood working as part of the team. When I registered, to begin with, I thought I'd like to have a home base on just one ward.

The first six months were ok, although it was a big leap from being a student to being a responsible, registered nurse. Nothing fully prepared me for the jump in responsibility to being a registrant. The buck stopped with me now. It was overwhelming at times. For three years I had worked under supervision, constantly asking questions, getting reassurance and checking things. Then there was no one to turn to. I was on my own. People were looking to me now!

In that first year of qualifying, I finished my preceptorship programme, which is a recommendation of the Nursing and Midwifery Council (NMC, 2020). I was in the last six months of a two-year rotation in renal medicine when I felt I had my first major wobble. I had been enjoying my job less and less over the last 18 months, feeling pressured when there weren't enough staff on shift. I was getting annoyed when I got moved to another ward, and then felt overwhelmed by just how much there was to do on a shift, plus constantly changing shift patterns. The hospital where I worked was huge, impersonal and not that friendly. I felt like a resource, just another grade on an off-duty rota, that could be moved from place to place like a pawn in a game of chess.

Although I rotated around the renal directorate, I began to feel bored and longed to be a student again. I really enjoyed being able to move to new specialties and learn new things, to work with no responsibility (I have perhaps blocked out the constant stress of having written assessments and having no money!). I missed my cohort, being with my friends, and I even missed going into uni – the place that had been my home, my social life, for three years. I began to think about leaving. I was wondering if I might be happier doing something else. As it all felt so impersonal, I did wonder, would the ward care if I left? Did I really make a difference? What would my quality of life be if I worked somewhere else that didn't have shifts, short staffing and huge responsibility?

I have always tried to keep fit – mainly by walking or going to the occassional gym class but when I started work as a registered nurse and began to feel overwhelmed, I thought a distraction might help, so I started running. I downloaded the 'Couch to 5k' app on my phone and really enjoyed it. I never thought of myself as a runner, or that I could run 5 kilometres – but I love it! I find that running three times a week – the days I go depend on my shifts – really helps keep my head straight. I feel so calm after a run and physically feel so much better. Running feels like 'me time', and it is so important for my well-being, for me – it works!

Elise's case study, although fictitious, is not such an unusual scenario and one that most of us can identify with and relate to. Retention is a particular problem with newly registered nursing staff and has been attributed to interrelated demographic factors such as age, years of experience, having children or dependents, all of which leads to job instability (Feixia Wu et al. 2022). It is suggested that newly registered healthcare professionals need higher levels of support than they perceive (Brook et al, 2024), which goes beyond preceptorship, and therefore is often not considered feasible, or indeed possible.

Elise also highlights the importance of physical exercise for well-being. Regular physical exercise can improve your mental health, mood and self-esteem, improve sleep and reduce chances of developing illness. Guidelines advise that adults should try to be active every day and aim for at least 150 minutes of physical activity each week. This can include walking or cycling as active travel, going to exercise classes or the gym or anything that increases your heart rate (NHS, 2021).

CRITICAL QUESTIONS

Explore the key issues in Elise's scenario as you answer the following questions.

- What emotional triggers is Elise likely to be experiencing?
- What role does the pressure of Elise's work, a sense of teamwork and feelings of self-worth and value have on any decision making?
- When would it be a suitable time to seek support and guidance in this scenario, and how might this be accessed?
- What might be the benefits to Elise and the organisation of undertaking a staff appraisal, or having access to some supervision?
- What other physical exercise could Elise engage with to enhance her sense of well-being?

Often retention issues appear to arise when managers are themselves too busy to have time to look out for and care for the individuals in the team that they work with. Encouraging staff to speak up about how they are experiencing their work environment, undertaking regular clinical supervision and annual appraisals might be some ways that give time to hear how staff are getting on, to be used as a way of spotting when and what types of support is needed. Many organisations provide discounted gym memberships, cycle to work incentives and well-being walking clubs, as well as free NHS resources to support physical activity and well-being – explore the many resources that are out there! NHS England made a pledge to improve working experiences for all staff in the organisation in its Peoples Promise (2020), aiming to better support its 1.3 million workforce. It signified a real commitment to staff.

CASE STUDY 2

Mark, an experienced occupational therapist, asks – can I see my future?

I initially gained an undergraduate degree in Psychology before completing a two-year occupational therapy pre-registration master's degree. The course was challenging to complete, but I learned a lot in a short space of time, attending a variety of placements, completing academic assignments and learning about research. Sharing the experiences throughout my training had been bonding for me and my small cohort. We were all from a variety of backgrounds and had different aspirations – but we were all in the same place and at the same time! Once we qualified, we had split apart to all work in different geographical areas.

I worked on a band 5 rotation in an acute hospital, before specialising as a band 6 in neurology which was community based. I really find the work interesting and rewarding but am beginning to feel 'stuck' with the day-to-day caseload. I wonder about what I can do to progress and continue learning. Working in the community setting is vastly different to the acute hospital. I am alone most of the time due to home visits and have much less clinical support than when I worked in the hospital. There is more responsibility, and I must make complex decisions quickly. I don't see how I can get a promotion, or what course I can do to help develop myself. I feel detached from my peers and a bit lost.

Always a keen bird watcher and longstanding member of the RSPB (Royal Society for the Protection of Birds), I now find this hobby an essential part of my well-being self-care package! I discovered mindfulness podcasts as my salvation through the tricky days at work. I use the NHS resources for the patients I see and for myself – practice what you preach! Trying to notice everyday things, keeping regular time to be mindful, trying something new, watching and naming thoughts and freeing myself from past worries has really helped my ability to cope with work stress issues. For me, mindfulness works. It keeps me level-headed and relaxed – which is how I like to be!

CRITICAL QUESTIONS

Explore the key issues in Mark's scenario as you answer the following questions.

- What might be the benefits for Mark in receiving clinical supervision?
- What might be the role of staff appraisal in Mark's future career trajectory?
- What role could social media play for Mark in accessing peer support in his current role?
- Where might Mark access further education opportunities, and what funding sources could be available?
- What other well-being strategies could Mark use to support his mental health?
- What is mindfulness, and does it work to support our mental well-being?

In Mark's scenario (as with Elise), the issues do not appear dissimilar. Feelings of being overwhelmed, isolated and undervalued start to create a negative narrative in the individual's mind that may make it seem pointless to reach out for help and advice. Employees' requirement needs are complex and must be met on many levels. Arguably the context that healthcare workers are currently exposed to are potentially compounding factors contributing to staff decisions whether or not to stay.

Mindfulness is practicing awareness of what is happening inside and outside of ourselves, including what is going on in our immediate environments and what we are feeling and thinking. This is beneficial as we become more self-aware of how we respond to stimuli, and we can recognise patterns in ourselves. Studies have shown that mindfulness can reduce stress, anxiety and depression. Mindfulness can be practiced as part of our everyday routine, for example whilst walking or eating (NHS, 2022).

REFLECTION 1

Before moving on to the next section relating to retention strategies, take a moment to complete one or all the following self-assessment quizzes to understand what may be currently impacting on your ability to both enjoy and feel valued in your current work environment.

- Get running with Couch to 5k: www.nhs.uk/live-well/exercise/get-running-with-couch-to-5k/
- NHS Breathing exercises for stress: www.nhs.uk/mental-health/self-help/guides-tools-and-activities/breathing-exercises-for-stress/
- MIND, Mindfulness exercises and tips: www.mind.org.uk/information-support/drugs-and-treatments/mindfulness/mindfulness-exercises-tips/
- NHS England Mindfulness resources www.england.nhs.uk/supporting-our-nhs-people/support-now/wellbeing-apps/
- NHS Mindfulness: www.nhs.uk/mental-health/self-help/tips-and-support/mindfulness/

SELF-ASSESSMENT QUIZZES

- NHS Check my Well-being – Self-assess your psychological and emotional well-being (leadershipacademy.nhs.uk): https://checkwellbeing.leadershipacademy.nhs.uk
- Keeping well a self-assessment: www.keepingwellnwl.nhs.uk/self-help-resources/self-assessment-questionnaires
- Better Health, Let's do this: How Are You? quiz (www.nhs.uk): www.nhs.uk/better-health/how-are-you-quiz/

CONTEXT

A professional healthcare workforce shortage is affecting health and social care provision on a global scale (WHO, 2015; Aslam et al, 2022). As populations continue to age, with increasing co-morbidity and associated complex care needs, a diminishing health and social care workforce will not be able to meet growing care needs (Kiplagat et al, 2022). Consequently, this workforce shortage raises considerable risk to long-term sustainable health and social and economic outcomes (Phuong et al, 2019).

Many staff are approaching retirement age or leaving their chosen profession early in pursuit of less stressful lifestyle options (Peterson et al, 2022; Shand et al, 2022), whilst in 2022/23, over 12,000 UK-registered nurses applied for a Certificate of Current Professional Status to register outside the UK, more than double the number the year before and four times more than in 2018/19 (Bazeer et al, 2024). A loss of health and social care staff has been intensified due to increased work pressures, being faced with elevated levels of influenza hospital admissions, an NHS backlog of routine work, further compounded by increased cost of living crisis, post-pandemic work-related trauma, deteriorating work conditions and an ongoing pay dispute (Boniol et al, 2022).

To address a continuing nursing workforce shortfall, the Conservative government, in its 2019 manifesto, pledged to increase nursing numbers by 50,000 and to achieve this number of nurses joining the register by March 2024 (Holmes and Maguire, 2022). The NHS Chief Nursing Officer reported in December 2023 that almost all (93 per cent) of the government's target of '50,000 more nurses' had been achieved through international recruitment. One in three nurses in the NHS in England have now been educated abroad (Bazeer et al, 2024).

Whilst nursing numbers are championed to be increasing, the number of vacancies held remains high, meaning the rate of recruitment is not having a meaningful impact on overall nursing staff workforce shortages and staff experiences at work. There remain widespread nurse shortages in the NHS, with 42,000 vacancies – or around one in nine posts – unfilled in September 2023. With the public sector financial restraints, these workforce shortages do not look to be addressed in the short term, despite the NHS Long Term Workforce Plan for further expansion (2023).

Balancing the number of new recruits to nursing from domestic nursing programmes with the outflow of nurses from those who leave employment, those who chose to work outside the health sector, retire or immigrate, all suggests a challenge to sustainability (State of the World's Nursing (SOWN), 2020). Health Education England (2017: 7) stresses 'the most cost-effective way to ensure the health and care system has the staff we need is to keep the people we already employ'. The need to retain nurses already working in healthcare is one approach, but it is important to also be mindful that for every nurse that leaves, there is an impact on the nurses who remain. As Buchan et al. (2022) note, the demand *for* nurses is putting demand *on* nurses, by increasing workloads and pressures.

The reasons why nurses leave is multiple. Ball et al. (2022) completed a scoping review on the retention of NHS nurses in 2021 and categorises the organisational factors causing nurses to leave into eight broad themes. Central to all retention factors is job satisfaction. Then there are other things such as work-life balance, relationships and support, achieving excellence in care, adequate staffing and resources, sense of control and being heard, opportunities to develop, pay and rewards; all are contributing factors to nurse attrition (Ball et al., 2022).

Dissatisfaction with their job drives many nurses to leave the profession. Equally, job satisfaction impacts on nurses' intention to stay (Pressley & Garside, 2023). Pressley and Garside (2023) describe job satisfaction occurs when an employee's needs are met, can overcome challenges and remain motivated. Job satisfaction is central to why nurses leave, yet as the figure shows, many other issues contribute to and interplay with it. Marufu et al, (2021) and Ball et al. (2022) agree that work-life balance;

pay and reward; standards of care; development opportunities; relationships, such as support from colleagues and managers; staffing levels; voice and control over working lives all play a vital part in the multiple factors that contribute to job satisfaction and why nurses leave. Pressley and Garside (2023) add that organisational commitment, organisational culture, emotional intelligence and stress management also contribute to experiences job satisfaction. In addition, demographic factors also impact on attrition, such as age, length of time in career and gender (Pressley & Garside, 2023).

For retention strategies to be effective, they need to take a comprehensive approach to staffing. No single intervention holds the promise to change retention of nurses. Both organisational and personal factors need to be considered since they both influence decisions to stay in the profession or leave. Retention interventions at an organizational level need to enhance the appeal of nursing whilst personal interventions can be utilized to improve well-being. Support for both interventions can have a positive impact on retention in the UK. Strategies that have demonstrated positive impact on retention are considered in the next section.

STRATEGIES TO ENCOURAGE STAFF TO REMAIN IN THEIR CHOSEN FIELD

Research has identified several factors that influence staff in health and social care to remain in their chosen fields. In a scoping review of retention of NHS nurses, Ball et al. (2022) organised these factors around the core theme of job satisfaction. Other reviews had similar findings, with additional emphasis on the impact of location and demographics (De Vries et al., 2023; Pressley and Garside, 2023). In this section, individual themes and strategies will be discussed.

OPPORTUNITIES FOR EDUCATION AND CAREER ADVANCEMENT

Lack of opportunities for education and career advancement is a factor in health and social care staff turnover at various career stages (Moseley et al., 2008; Marufu et al., 2021; De Vries et al., 2023; Brook et al., 2024). Successful strategies include clinical ladder programmes, where financial and promotional rewards are given for engagement with leadership and education programmes (Drenkard and Swartwout, 2005). What you can do:

- Be proactive in seeking out learning opportunities and funding streams for skills development.
- Identify meaningful goals and career pathways, and steps needed to achieve these.
- At interview, ask about opportunities for education and career advancement.

SUPPORTIVE LEADERSHIP AND MANAGEMENT

Leadership and management are a key component in health and social care job satisfaction. High staff turnover has been associated with lack of support from managers, staff not feeling recognised or valued, lack of communication about organisational factors and feeling powerless with their organisational input (Cowden et al., 2011; Marufu et al., 2021). What you can do:

- Engage in opportunities to contribute your opinion and influence on the wider organisation through meetings, committees, surveys or taking on a 'champion' role.
- Leadership exists at all levels – be aware of your own leadership ability and how to develop this.

SUPPORTIVE WORKPLACE CULTURE

Workplace culture has been strongly linked with employee well-being and retention. Creating a positive, supportive culture is the responsibility of everyone. The actions, words and attitudes of employees at all levels influence group cohesion and dynamics. Positive support including peer support and interpersonal relationships have been associated with lower turnover (Bae, 2024). However negative social cultures such as racism and discrimination (Pressley & Garside, 2023) and incivility (D'Ambra & Andrews, 2014) impact negatively on staff well-being and aspirations. What you can do:

- Be aware of your own behaviour and how this affects others.
- Set an example to others through your behaviours and actions.
- Show support and understanding to students and colleagues, including international staff.
- Have a zero-tolerance approach to discrimination or bullying.

ADEQUATE STAFFING LEVELS

Working in an understaffed team can be a challenge. In this situation it is vital that we support each other, with teamwork being more important than ever. What you can do:

- Be patient and kind to students and agency staff – this helps the bigger retention picture.
- Check with your local workforce plans, and also undertake a safer staffing checklist, which can be found via your union, or on the NHS England website: www.england.nhs.uk/nursingmidwifery/safer-staffing-nursing-and-midwifery/.

- The Royal College of Nursing has also identified some workforce standards and resources that can be found via their website: www.rcn.org.uk/Professional-Development/Nursing-Workforce-Standards.

SUPPORT FOR NEWLY QUALIFIED STAFF

Newly qualified health and social care professionals benefit from increased practical and emotional support, to help with the transition from student to independent practitioner. Research has demonstrated that mentorship and preceptorship programmes have a positive effect on staff well-being and retention (Halter et al, 2017). What you can do:

- Be kind and supportive to new starters. Give them time to develop their confidence.
- Enable new starters to identify own learning needs and take responsibility for achieving goals.

Consider what further support newly qualified staff might require, such as legacy practitioner engagement or coaching and mentoring post any preceptorship period. The NHS England site has more information on Legacy Mentor roles: www.england.nhs.uk/looking-after-our-people/supporting-people-in-early-and-late-career/legacy-mentoring/.

MENOPAUSE SUPPORT

As a largely female workforce, 19 per cent of the total NHS workforce are experiencing or approaching menopause (The Strategy Unit, 2023). Symptoms include brain fog, memory loss, feeling overwhelmed, loss of confidence, work performance, absenteeism and retention. NHS England has recognised the impact of menopause on employees' health and well-being, and provided guidance and resources to organisations (NHS England, 2022). What you can do:

- Complete the 30-minute NHS Menopause Awareness e-learning.
- Be mindful of symptoms that may be affecting yourself or colleagues.

WELL-BEING

Looking after our physical and mental health has a direct correlation with how we feel each day, in and out of work. Personal qualities of self-awareness, self-efficacy, resilience and understanding of self has been linked with workplace retention (Joseph et al., 2022), as has health status including sleep and healthy lifestyles (Bae, 2023).

What you can do is consider the following:

- Be aware of your own triggers and stressors.
- Reflect on demanding situations, and use this to build resilience.
- Take an annual leave regularly.
- Use breaktimes well – get away from screens, spend time outdoors, refuel and hydrate.
- Utilise well-being services offered by the employer.
- Talk to friends, family and colleagues.
- Have hobbies outside of work.
- Look after yourself through a healthy diet, exercise and sleep routine.
- Be kind to yourself.
- Learn from mistakes.

FINANCIAL RENUMERATION, BENEFITS AND RECOGNITION

Recognition of employees' contributions to the workplace has been linked with improved staff retention through financial awards, employee benefits and praise (Moseley et al, 2008; Williamson et al, 2022).

What you can do:

- Think about promotion opportunities and pay increments when looking for jobs.
- Look at your employee pension and plan to top this up, or open a private pension for when you want to/can retire.

REFLECTION TASK 2

Having read the earlier strategies relating to retention, now is the time for action. Use one or both of the following toolkits to explore your own career/employment needs in more detail, including the changes and support you need both inside and outside the work environment. Develop your own immediate short-term and long-term strategies to enable you to stay fulfilled at work.

- The North Kent Training Hub offers a Stay and Grow Conversations toolkit and templates (northkenttraininghub.nhs.uk): www.northkenttraininghub.nhs.uk/post/stay-and-grow-conversations-toolkit-and-templates.
- Lots of advice and bite size information and resources via the NHS website Live Well – NHS: www.nhs.uk/live-well/.

- When looking for your next employer what matters most to you? Culture, total rewards, rates of pay, location?
- Write a 'must have' list that you can use as a checklist when you are next looking for a new post.
- Have practice interviews, share your CV with a trusted colleague for feedback and think about what questions you wish to ask of your potential new employers at the interview. Read their strategy documents and tailor questions about your future development and explain how you bring your specific strengths to the role, in achieving their strategic vision.

IN SUMMARY

This chapter has demonstrated that embarking on a healthcare career is a journey of continuous learning, personal growth and professional development. From the initial steps as a novice, brimming with enthusiasm yet facing the complexities of healthcare, to the seasoned expert who navigates challenging situations with confidence and wisdom, the path is often both rewarding and demanding. Most health and social care professionals have long, successful careers; looking after your own health and being aware of your professional needs can aid this.

Staying in the game is important to us as individuals and to the wider population. A sense of belonging is central to retention, and the feeling that one is valued and has a key place in an organisation cannot be underestimated. Many of the strategies presented stem from enhancing this sense of belonging. We all meet challenges, and we all need support at different points of our careers. Make use of the many resources available to help you stay. A selection of further reading is presented subsequently to enable you to visit lessons learned by others and explore your own strategies for staying in the game.

FURTHER READING

- **Personal growth stories** in nursing highlight the vulnerabilities, the mistakes and the invaluable lessons learned during the early days of a career in nursing. These narratives highlight individual nurses' personal and professional growth and serve as a source of encouragement and guidance for others at various stages of their nursing careers.
  From Novice to Expert: Personal Growth Stories in Nursing (rnnet.org)
- **The Mental Health Foundation** website has a section on work-life balance and offers very practical tips for achieving a sensible work-life balance alongside many other useful resources related to protecting your mental health.
  www.mentalhealth.org.uk/explore-mental-health/a-z-topics/work-life-balance

- **The Royal College of Nursing** has some helpful toolkits on how to identify external and internal work-based pressures, raise issues informally and escalate if necessary. Problems at work checklist | Royal College of Nursing (rcn. org.uk).
- **Wilkinson's (2021)** *Nurse burnout: A caregiver's guide to stress management and building resilience in healthcare: Relieving stress with mindfulness, meditation, and coping strategies*. This useful guidebook is applicable to any healthcare professional who is experiencing stress, anxiety and lack of resilience.
- **Appraisals and performance reviews: how to prepare (RCN).** Constructive meetings give you the opportunity to discuss your achievements, challenges and expectations. They also allow you to raise any issues outside of your control that might impact on your performance, such as staffing levels or system failures. Appraisals and performance reviews: a checklist to help you prepare | Royal College of Nursing (rcn.org.uk).
- **The principles of preceptorship (NMC 2020)** Access this guidance to understand the benefits of preceptorship for you. Its main aim is help you integrate as a newly registered professional into your new team and place of work. Preceptorship is not designed to replace appraisals, be a substitute for a formal induction or mandatory training. Principles of preceptorship – the Nursing and Midwifery Council (nmc.org.uk).

REFERENCES

Aslam, M. Z., Trail, M., Cassell, III A. K., Khan A. B. and Payne, S (2022) Establishing a sustainable healthcare environment in low-and middle-income countries. *British Journal of Urology International*, 129 (2), 134–142.

Bae S. H. (2023) Comprehensive assessment of factors contributing to the actual turnover of newly licensed registered nurses working in acute care hospitals: A systematic review. *BMC Nursing*, 22(1), 31.

Bae S. H. (2024) Assessing the impacts of nurse staffing and work schedules on nurse turnover: A systematic review. *International Nursing Review*, 71(1), 168–179.

Ball J., Ejebu O. Z. and Saville C. (2022) What keeps nurses in nursing? A scoping review into nurse retention. *Nursing Times*, 118(11), 40–1.

Bazeer N., Kelly L. and Buchan J. (2024) *Nursing locally, thinking globally: UK-registered nurses and their intentions to leave*. The Health Foundation. (accessed 8 May 2024).

Boniol M., Kunjumen T., Nair T. S., Siyam A., Campbell J. and Diallo, K. (2022) The global health workforce stock and distribution in 2020 and 2030: A threat to equity and 'universal' health coverage? *BMJ Global Health*, 7(6), e009316.

Brook J., Aitken L. and Salmon D. (2024) Effectiveness appraisal of interventions to increase retention of newly qualified nurses implemented in the final year of pre-registration programmes: A literature review. *Nurse Education in Practice*, 74, 103851.

Buchan J., Catton H. and Shaffer F. (2022) *Sustain and retain in 2022 and beyond*. International Centre on Nurse Migration. Philadelphia. www.icn.ch/sites/default/files/2023-04/Sustain%

20and%20Retain%20in%202022%20and%20Beyond-%20The%20global%20nursing%20workforce%20and%20the%20COVID-19%20pandemic.pdf (accessed 13 June 2024).

Cowden T., Cummings G. and Profetto-McGrath J. (2011) Leadership practices and staff nurses' intent to stay: A systematic review. *Journal of Nursing Management*, 19(4), 461–477.

D'ambra A. and Andrews D. (2014) Incivility, retention and new graduate nurses: an integrated review of the literature. *Journal of Nursing Management*, 22(6), 735–742.

De Vries N., Boone A., Godderis L., Bouman J., Szemik S., Matranga D. and de Winter P (2023) The race to retain healthcare workers: A systematic review on factors that impact retention of nurses and physicians in hospitals. *Inquiry: The Journal of Health Care Organization, Provision, and Financing*, 60

Drenkard, K. and Swartwout, E. (2005) Effectiveness of a clinical ladder program. *Journal of Nursing*. https://doi.org/10.1097/00005110–200511000–00007.

Feixia Wu, Yuewen Lao, Ying Feng, Jiaqing Zhu, Yating Zhang. and Liuyan Li (2022) Worldwide prevalence and associated factors of nursing staff turnover: A systematic review and meta-analysis. *Nursing Open*. www.ncbi.nlm.nih.gov/pmc/articles/PMC10802134/pdf/NOP2-11-e2097.pdf (accessed 13 June 2024).

Glogowska M., Young P. and Lockyer L. (2007) Should I go, or should I stay? A study of factors influencing students' decisions on early leaving. *Active Learning in Higher Education*, 8(1), 63–77.

Halter M., Pelone F., Boiko O., Beighton C., Harris R., Gale J., Gourlay S. and Drennan V. (2017) Interventions to reduce adult nursing turnover: A systematic review of systematic reviews. *The Open Nursing Journal*, 11, 108–123.

Health Education England. (2017) *Facing the Facts, Shaping the Future, A health and care workforce strategy for England to 2027*. www.hee.nhs.uk/sites/default/files/documents/Facing%20the%20Facts,%20Shaping%20the%20Future%20%E2%80%93%20a%20draft%20health%20and%20care%20workforce%20strategy%20for%20England%20to%202027.pdf (accessed 13 June 2024).

Holmes J. and Maguire, D. (2022) *Is the NHS on track to recruit 50,000 more nurses? Hitting the target but missing the point*. April 2022. www. kingsfund.org.uk/blog/2022/04/nhs-recruit-50000-more-nurses (accessed 5 April 2024).

Joseph B., Jacob S., Lam L. and Rahman M. A. (2022) Factors influencing the transition and retention of mental health nurses during the initial years of practice: Scoping review. *Journal of Nursing Management*, 30(8), 4274–4284.

Kiplagat J., Tran D. N., Barber T., Njuguna B., Vedanthan R., Triant V. A. and Pastakia S. D. (2022) How health systems can adapt to a population ageing with HIV and comorbid disease. *The Lancet HIV*, 9(4), 281–292.

Marufu T., Collins A., Vargas L., Gillespie L. and Almghairbi D. (2021) Factors influencing retention among hospital nurses: Systematic review. *British Journal of Nursing*, 30(5), 302–308.

Moseley A., Jeffers L. and Paterson J. (2008) The retention of the older nursing workforce: a literature review exploring factors which influence the retention and turnover of older nurses. *Contemporary Nurse: A Journal for the Australian Nursing Profession*, 30(1), 46–56.

NHS. (2021) Benefits of Exercise. Available at: Benefits of exercise – NHS (www.nhs.uk) (accessed 01 July 2024)

NHS. (2022) Mindfulness. Available at: Mindfulness – NHS (www.nhs.uk). (accessed 01 July 2024)

NHS England. (2020) Our NHS People Promise. Available at: NHS England" Our NHS People Promise. (accessed 03 July 2024)

NHS England. (2022) *Supporting our NHS people through menopause: Guidance for line managers and colleagues*. Available at: www.england.nhs.uk/publication/supporting-our-nhs-people-through-menopause-guidance-for-line-managers-and-colleagues/ (accessed 20 May 2024).

Nursing and Midwifery Council. (2020) Principle of Preceptorship Principles of preceptorship – The Nursing and Midwifery Council (nmc.org.uk) (accessed 17 June 2024).

Peterson C. J., Lee B. and Nugent K. (2022) COVID-19 vaccination hesitancy among healthcare workers – A review. *Vaccines*, *10*(6), 948.

Phuong J. M., Penm J., Chaar B., Oldfield L. D. and Moles R. (2019) The impacts of medication shortages on patient outcomes: A scoping review. *PloS One*, *14*(5). https://journals.plos.org/plosone/article?id=10.1371/journal.pone.0215837 (accessed 13 June 2024).

Pressley C. and Garside J. (2023) Safeguarding the retention of nurses: A systematic review on determinants of nurse's intentions to stay. *Nursing Open*, 10(5), 2842–2858.

Shand R., Parker S., Liddle J., Spolander G., Warwick L. and Ainsworth S. (2022) After the applause: Understanding public management and public service ethos in the fight against Covid-19. *Public Management Review*, 1–23.

State of the World's Nursing (SOWN). (2020) *Investing in education, jobs and leadership*. World Health Organisation. www.who.int/publications/i/item/9789240003279 (accessed 13 June 2024).

The Strategy Unit. (2023) *Menopause and the NHS workforce*. Available at: www.strategyunitwm.nhs.uk/publications/menopause-and-nhs-workforce (accessed 20 May 2024).

Wilkinson N. K. (2021) *Nurse Burnout: A Caregiver's Guide to Stress Management and Building Resilience in Healthcare: Relieving Stress with Mindfulness, Meditation, and Coping Strategies*. Kindle.

Williamson L., Burog W. and Taylor R. (2022) A scoping review of strategies used to recruit and retain nurses in the health care workforce. *Journal of Nursing Management*, 30(7): 2845–2853.

World Health Organisation. (2015) *Health workforce and services: Draft global strategy on human resources for health: Workforce 2030*. Rep. Secr. Exec. Board EB13836 Available at: http://apps.who.int/gb/ebwha/pdf_files/EB138/B138_36-en.pdf (accessed 2 April 2024).

Chapter 10

Eat, drink and be merry; tomorrow we diet

Sally Hardy

INTRODUCTION

'How healthy are the health care staff?' Bolton et al.'s (2024) article title posed this question, which helped me rethink what this chapter can offer. As health and social care staff, our focus is to ensure others can remain healthy and recover from being ill, or from traumatic health experiences. We aim to heal others, not just as health promotional educators, health prevention seekers and health care service brokers for our patients, communities and populations but also in how to pass on our knowledge. But there is the issue. When do we consider our own health and well-being as a priority?

Bolton et al, (2024) reports that diet, physical activity, sleep patterns and psychological distress are all indicators of quality well-being. Our waist circumference, eating and physical habits, all can lead to future chronic health problems, such as diabetes and cardiovascular and musculoskeletal deteriorations. Health care staff are known to have low healthy compliance, in terms of eating well, alcohol consumption and physical activity recommendations (Gifkins et al., 2018; Schneider et al., 2019; Kagan et al., 2022; Bolton et al., 2024).

Integral to healthy living is mental well-being. Greater emphasis is recognised in the need to seek a balance between mind and body, as a core and essential component to health and well-being (Sharma et al., 2024). Feeling well and seeking happiness has become a multimillion-pound global industry. There are more well-being apps available on the market than any other. An artificial intelligence (AI) revolution is changing the face of mental health treatments and gathering latest trends in promoting well-being. According to Business of Apps (2025) website, wellness related apps generated equivalent to £740 million in 2023, with over 50

DOI: 10.4324/9781041057956-11

million people using wellness apps. North America spent the most on wellness apps, followed by Europe, then Asia Pacific regions.

In this chapter I aim to outline what we know to be useful, as bite-size pieces of information from which to fuel our minds and bodies. It is how we approach eating, drinking and living 'merry' lives that will influence our choices and address long-term healthier ways of living.

CASE STUDY

Working 12-hour shifts was playing havoc with my love life. How on earth can I get to feel and look good when I have been running around all day looking after patients, cheering up my colleagues, skipping meal breaks to deal with a mountain of paperwork before I can down tools and go home to get ready to go out again. Then, because I had no energy left, I end up sitting in front of the telly, snacking on crisps, chocolates and wine, which is about my cooking tolerance limit, especially when it's dark and cold outside. This was the pattern of my life, until I had a serious issue with my health.

I had a stroke. I woke up with a weak sensation all down my left side, which made me feel I was still drunk. I managed to call my neighbour, who lives downstairs in the same block, and got them to come up and check on me. They called an ambulance immediately when they saw the state of me.

Several weeks later, I am being pushed to and from exercise class with the physiotherapist to rebuild my muscle strength. Slowly my speech is returning, which is a huge relief. It is the fine motor skills I still have trouble with, especially doing up small buttons on my clothes. I get so angry and frustrated and am very easily tired by simple tasks. But I am one of the lucky ones. The doctor said because I haven't smoked, I saved myself a whole series of worse scenarios in my recovery time and rehabilitation journey.

Occupational therapy sessions have had me drawing. I didn't realise how much pleasure you can get from really looking at something and putting your own unique version of it down on paper. I've even tried my shacking hands at printing. Then once I got more confident I recently achieved some lino-cutting which I never knew was a thing, but now I lose myself in the finer details, carving out the images, which again is helping get my hand-eye coordination back.

Yoga has also come into my life as I continue to work on my health now that I have been discharged home. At first I went to a swimming class referred by the hospital. But now I find yoga is my go-to form of exercise. Those gentle movements of stretching, positioning and holding poses, learning how to breathe deeply into my lungs, through my nostrils, one by one. Humming, chanting. I am almost a hippie. I am eating more pulses and vegetables too!

What have I learned from this whole experience? It is never too late to start looking after ourselves. Keeping active, mentally and physically, is so important. I am about to go back to work and have missed everyone these past long six months. Everyone has been so supportive during my absence. But I needed to change my habits. I know that now. I also know I have to keep this up if I want to avoid another more damaging health event further down the line.

CRITICAL QUESTIONS

- Reading through the case study, what aspects of your lifestyle patterns can you relate to it?
- What do you do to stimulate yourself to making healthy choices, whether about your physical or your mental agility?
- Are you worried about your, or someone else's, physical health and mental well-being?

REFLECTION

1. Write down a list of things you do regularly, and at what time of day.
2. Mark off which ones are for your physical health and which ones help your mental well-being.
3. Then grade these in terms of highly effective, and those that are less so.
4. How many do you have leaning towards which end of the spectrum (good or bad habits)?
5. Where can you improve your physical and mental fitness?
6. Identify what your goals are to address some of these habits.
7. Then set yourself goals for achieving these improvements. Be realistic.

8. Who can support you to make these more healthy routines become a new habit?
9. What timeline are you giving yourself to get started?

HEALTHY LIVING

Research from a 75-year study of human development commenced in 1938 has identified that loneliness kills. In comparison, it is those who have good social connections who are happier and live longer, healthier lives. So, is it true that what we eat, drink and seek for our happiness are all important components of living well? Having healthy relationships is what appears to be a significant buffer to life's tragedies and traumas. 'Being in a secure and protective relationship appears to help us stay sharper longer. Not just physically, but also our brains' (Waldinger, 2016; Ted Talk).

EATING (B)

We probably all know too well that healthy foods are those that contain natural ingredients – nutrients, vitamins and minerals that feed our brain and bodies, plus influence gut microbes, which in turn help us feel physically and emotionally well. If you focus on buying and cooking with seasonal fruits and vegetables throughout the year, you will be feeding your body all the minerals, vitamins and variety of nutrients it needs, as natural foods contain antioxidants and nutrients that support a healthy heart and healthy mind. Have you ever thought that summer fruits and vegetables have higher water content and carotenoids that helps us manage the heat of the sun when at its highest? Then winter vegetables have higher starch levels, often dark rich colours that provide energy to help keep us warm whilst the sun is at its lowest.

Avoiding processed foods can help reduce inflammation and other chronic health conditions, as our bodies work hard to rid itself of unnecessarily high amounts of 'toxins', those elements our bodies cannot tolerate in high levels. Processed foods are readily available to buy, because they can be stored for longer. Yet to achieve this, they have been highly processed with additional chemical substances added in high doses, such as modified starch, artificial sweeteners, flavourings (e.g. monosodium glutamate), colourants, saturated fats, hydrolysed proteins and bulking agents, such as foams and gels. In comparison, we need to be eating more whole foods, such as wholegrains, fruit, vegetables, meat, poultry, fish, eggs, nuts, seeds, herbs and spices. Organic food sources work to reduce the amount of chemicals sprayed or contained within the soil in which our food grows. Choosing organic produce where possible will give back to the soil and help us feed our future generations, whilst also promoting healthy soil, although they can have a higher price tag as a result.

How do we swap out the convenient, readily available, colourfully packaged and appealing processed foods for more natural ingredients? There is an NHS website that offers a series of healthy swaps to give people ideas for how to deal with 'hangry', busy, fussy families. The notion of food 'swap while you shop' is to replace high-sugar, salty foods with those still readily available and appealing. Checking food labels that use the traffic light system, replacing meals that have higher green than red or amber labels on the packaging, will cut down the salts and sugars whilst still ensuring you are getting familiar family favourites. Gradually replacing sugary breakfast cereals with fruits, nuts and plain yoghurt, or porridge, will take time. But worth a try at least once a week for starters, introducing replacement or swaps.

The late Michael Mosley (2023/2024) spoke of 'just one thing' in his series of television and radio programmes to help people with managing the swap to making healthy choices. From eating more slowly, to brushing your teeth standing on one foot for two minutes. His discussions with knowledge experts offer an entertaining and revealing insight into what we can do as small steps towards improved health and well-being.

DRINKING

Drinking water has always been seen as a major health benefit, a vital life source (Kleiner, 1999). We can survive only days without water, but weeks without food. Our bodies have high level of water content (50–75 per cent) compared to a cucumber that has 96 per cent water content. Our mental capacity is also affected by how hydrated we are, with studies being undertaken to ensure health care staff, particularly during their 12-hour shifts, have access to drinking water; otherwise their decision making and health can be effected (Alozmar et al., 2013). Yet that research did not stop or prevent nurses from having access denied to their personal drinking water bottles on shift as an infection control risk (Devereux, 2022).

Becoming dehydrated can be a side effect of high alcohol intake, as alcohol is a diuretic (Shirreffs and Maughan, 1997). Urinating high sodium and potassium after drinking alcohol affects kidney, brain and liver function, making us more highly susceptible to damaging these organs over time. Ensuring water is drunk to quench thirst, both before and after drinking alcohol, does something towards restoring electrolyte balance; but most often, drinking alcohol leads to wanting to sleep and waking up with a headache due to being dehydrated. The body can only process blood alcohol content one standard drink per hour. Therefore, the quicker you drink, the higher blood alcohol content (BAC), which will take your body longer to process and get rid of, either via your kidneys (urination) or liver (blood).

In America, alcohol disorder affects 29 million people and causes over 140,000 deaths per year (Koob, 2024). In the UK there has been a 400% rise in liver-related mortalities in the past three decades (Subhani et al., 2024). If you are drinking alcohol every day and cannot go without a drink at least two consecutive days a week, this is identified as low-level dependence. Risky alcohol consumption is identified as 17 standard drink units (SDUs) per week, or 2–2.5 SDUs per day for women and 4 SDUs for men (Pérula-Jiménez et al, 2024).

Heavy drinking and mental health issues are linked, yet we do not often recognise how these are closely interlinked (Jackson et al., 2023). Jackson et al. (2023) conclude that more often than not, it is a person's relational and social situation that provides the best indicator of their health status. Seeking to treat underlying rationale for harmful behaviours, is often overlooked in health and care service offer, which focuses on presenting symptom relief. Most of our patterns of behaviour when it comes to healthy life choices arise from addictions, which in turn provides an opportunity to use evidence-based behavioural health treatments and non-pharmacological interventions.

BEING 'MERRY'

Understanding well-being and what makes us happy has been seen as an indicator and measure of a person's overall health, success and functioning. Traditional well-being measures have focused on life satisfaction or happiness per se, whilst other measures use a single item measure of subjective well-being, which do not have high levels of reliability (Cummins et al., 2003; Lau et al., 2005; Huppert et al., 2009). For this reason, measurement requires sensitivity that captures transient aspects of positive and negative responses to well-being. Such a holistic approach to being healthy is moving towards interest in how to emphasise transient states of happiness, with a goal of providing sustainable well-being over time.

Well-being is complex and can depend on the way a person interacts with others, understands and responds to, or with, their environmental circumstances (Gray and Tischler, 2024). There is growing interest and evidence that social contribution, such as volunteering or doing things for others, contributes to both physical and mental health (Meier and Stutzer, 2008; Nichol et al., 2024). Gender and age also need to be taken into consideration and remains an important area of research, as the variety of relationships between age and well-being becomes better understood.

In commonly used well-being instruments, these usually capture some health dimensions; yet, it is widely recognised there are additional, non-health dimensions that need to be included. These are broadly classified into four main well-being concepts that seek to capture aspects of a person's

1. purpose in life and achievement (wishes, goals, values, spirituality, self-realisation, activity level, achievements, work);
2. worries about security and safety (present and future);
3. financial well-being (money, financial situation, standard of living); and
4. personal freedom (control, autonomy, independence).

Less frequently mentioned in well-being research are dimensions related to capturing aspects of what constitutes pleasure, engaging in creativity and play, or how well-being can be related to a person's physical environment such as where they live, their community and neighbourhood and access to nature, as either green or blue spaces (Tate et al, 2024).

The Department of Health's Boorman review (Boorman, 2010) specifically addressed the health and well-being at work of healthcare staff. It highlighted the need for a whole-system interventions approach, which incorporates input from staff regarding their local needs and contexts alongside involvement of management staff at all levels of the organisation. The review proposed five system-level changes for healthcare workplaces to improve staff health and well-being: understanding local staff needs, staff engagement at all levels, strong visible leadership, support for health and well-being at senior management and board level and a focus on management capability and capacity to improve staff health and well-being. In the United Kingdom, these healthcare workplace improvement plans are supported by the National Institute for Health and Care Excellence (NICE) incorporated into the NHS Health and Well-being Improvement Framework (2011).

Brand et al.'s (2017) study into what interventions improve healthcare staff's health and well-being focused on supporting or improving individual coping and personal resilience skills, rather than what is affecting the wider components of the workplace environemnt. They concluded there was still a paucity of information available to report which approach was proving most effective. However, post pandemic, emphasis is still being placed on aspects of workplace well-being, with employers taking greater responsibility for introducing policies and procedures that can promote and sustain healthier behaviours amongst their workforce in an attempt to address the high levels of long-term sickness and absence found in the health and care workforce (Minshall et al, 2024).

TOMORROW WE DIET

We cannot wait until tomorrow before we change our habits. Our water, soils, air and landscape are all polluted by years of chemical and industrial usage. Swapping out aerosol sprays, deodorants and cleaning liquids can make a small difference in terms of your shopping habits but can also impact air and water pollution over time. Seeing the particles in the air when you travel under tunnels and look up at the soot blackening the roof and walls, do you begin to realise how much our air is harmful, risking damage to our respiratory organs? Green plants and trees are playing a major part in keeping our cities cooler and air cleaner.

A growing awareness of the impact of climate change on our health and well-being has led to a whole new diagnosis of 'climate anxiety'. Axatova and Axatova's (2024) study identified that engaging in eco-friendly habits, such as recycling to reduce waste, utilising renewable energy, increasing our time seeking out being in green or blue spaces, can make a huge difference to air quality, and water security, which in turn improves our mental health and well-being. We recognise that continuation of human and animal life depends on the behaviours, policies and practices of mankind today.

Being sustainable is based on the principle of ensuring we limit disturbance to our planets ecosystem and, if anything, attempting to reduce harm to rebalance nature's ability to heal. Therefore, this chapter is actually all about our responsibility to all our futures. Attempting to eat well and focusing on the most sustainable and natural sources of foods all help in addressing our impact on the environment within which we live and work.

CONCLUSION: LIVING A SUSTAINABLE LIFE

Today, I will do one small task that will contribute toward the achievement of a life goal.

(Casey, 2022: Jan 5)

Many spend their lives seeking happiness through wealth and career success. Only to find that when older age and ill-health catches us, striving for these things has not necessarily brought the inner peace and wellness we were after, after all. Richard Rohr (2023) talks about falling upwards in the latter stages of life; once the climb up the career ladder has been reached, where do we go next?

Osteen (2024) lists seven steps to living up to our full potential. These are to, first, enlarge your vision, then develop a healthy self-image, discover the power of your thoughts and words, let go of the past, find strength in adversity, live to give and, finally, choose to be happy. French philosopher Pascal states that our problems all stem from our inability to sit quietly and alone (Casey, 2022).

Whatever you have taken from this chapter, or indeed from the entire book, please understand I and many of the authors are not writing as health freaks, or fitness and well-being gurus, nutritionists or saints. But we write from personal and professional experiences, based on our own life's interesting twist and turns. We all make mistakes, experience heartache. I have often sought refuge in food and wine. Yet, knowing where and how I can make a difference has led me to constantly seek healthier options in my choices, so that I can continue to inform, share, live and laugh together with others along the way.

We each remain responsible for our own choices. Even down to how we react and respond to others who might wish to judge or criticise us. Taking accountability for our actions, and the consequences associated with these choices, is one path to self-awareness, acceptance and peace of mind. Set yourself a goal. Work with those who share your vision and values. Fuel your mind and your body with life's good things.

All the best in your exploration of healthy living, eating, drinking and being merry.

LEARNING RESOURCES

Try working through the alphabet to a healthier lifestyle. I have developed one here for you. Try and build one of your own. Maybe get the whole family involved:

Activate your inner eco-warrior
Be kind
Care for the environment

Drink litres of water each day

Eat and drink with a plan

Focus on fresh fruit and seasonal veggies

Get out into nature

Honey is the most natural form of sugar

Invest in you

Junk food is bad, so swap it for healthier treats

Know what works for you (see STRENGTH model later)

Learn a new skill

Monitor alcohol intake

Notice calorific value in foods

Organise your day to include increased activity

Prepare meal plans and shopping to a set budget

Recognise your sleep habits and need for rest

Seek advice and help as needed

Treat yourself and family occasionally

Upcycle clothes and waste products

Vitamin supplements are not necessary when eating a varied diet

Weekends and downtime are important

X: Extinction lists are growing, notice what and how your garden or window shelf can help

Young at heart allows for optimism and a willingness to try new things

Zen practices, such as yoga, mindfulness and meditation

Table 10.1 is based on Brown's (2022) STRENGTH mnemonic, offering eight ways to motivate yourself towards improvements.

Go back to the reflective task and see if this table can help create your own well-being plan.

FURTHER READING

MIND has a whole series of interesting materials on improving your mental well-being, from journaling, stress reduction, connecting with others and help with sleep.

www.mind.org.uk/information-support/tips-for-everyday-living/wellbeing/

The British Heart Foundation has a series of useful tips relating to activity, nutrition and well-being. Visit their website for more information.

www.bhf.org.uk/informationsupport/heart-matters-magazine/wellbeing/how-to-motivate-yourself-to-get-healthy

Table 10.1 Brown's STRENGTH mnemonic for healthy living

Strength	How	Why	What
Self-determination	*Do it your way.*	Autonomy is an important aspect of any behaviour change; feeling in control of decisions helps improve confidence.	Select from a choice of healthy options available, to find what suits you and brings you satisfaction.
Technique	*Do it well.*	A desire to master, or get good at, something, known as performance incentive, brings additional motivations. As we see and feel benefits, our capability and confidence rise, as well as the desire to share that experience with others.	Choose what you want to get good at, whether it is vegetarian cooking, a new sport, craft or any other self-determined healthy practice.
Relatedness	*Do it together.*	Being socially connected and valued by others is an important element to well-being. Support groups and peer encouragement have proven important for long-term sustainable health behaviour changes.	Get your friends and family involved in your new pursuits and interests in being healthy. Book into a class, so new friendship and social groups can be built. Plus, a sense of not wanting to let others down might be a motivator to ensure you turn up to class each week.
External awareness	*Understand your circumstances.*	Identifying what you can control and what you cannot will allow your positive decisions towards health improvement to become more meaningful and achievable.	Asking for help is not a weakness. Recognising where others can support and encourage you is an important step in realising potentials.

(Continued)

Table 10.1 (Continued)

Strength	How	Why	What
Novelty	*Mix it up.*	Some people love a routine, whilst others find motivation through trying something new. If you are someone who needs stimulation, then try something new.	Seeking out new and novel ways to contribute to your recipes exercise regimen or daily habits can keep energy levels high and prevent boredom from setting in and those initial motivations from fading away.
Goal setting	*Set clear, rewarding goals*	How you set appropriate, realistic goals is important to determining whether or not you can achieve them. Intrinsic goals, are ones that bring enjoyment, in what you are doing and why.	Choose activities that bring you joy, choose foods or activities that you enjoy. See healthy choices as pleasurable, rather than a punishment. Keep your eye on the prize, of feeling more energised and your clothes fitting more comfortably.
Tenacity	*Be tenacious.*	A key ingredient for success is to keep trying despite some inevitable challenges. Being tenacious requires a commitment to self, and is a good indication for achieving realistic goals.	Recognising at the outset that this is a long-term, not short-term, activity. Sticking with it and overcoming hurdles bring a sense of personal achievement and is a good sign of leadership potential.
Honesty	*Be truthful.*	The ability to be honest with yourself and with others is about knowing our characteristics and traits. Being honest will help in your pursuit of a healthy life.	Knowing what and how you overcome challenges will ensure you recognise what supports and enables your success.

REFERENCES

Alozmar, M. Z., Akkam, A., Alashqar, S. and Eldali, A. (2013). Decreased hydration status of emergency department physicians and nurses by the end of their shift. *International journal of emergency medicine, 6*(1), 27.

Axatova, D. and Axatova, X. (2024). Integrating ecology and healthy living: Strategies for sustainable wellness. *E3S Web of Conferences, 587*, 02015. EDP Sciences.

Bolton, K. A., Fraser, P., Allender, S., Fitzgerald, R. and Brumby, S. (2024) How healthy are the healthcare staff in a rural health service? A cross-sectional study. *International Journal of Nursing Studies Advances, 6*, 100186.

Boorman, S. (2010). Health and well-being of the NHS workforce. *Journal of Public Mental Health, 9*(1), 4–7.

Brand, S. L., Thompson Coon, J., Fleming, L. E., Carroll, L., Bethel, A. and Wyatt, K. (2017). Whole-system approaches to improving the health and wellbeing of healthcare workers: A systematic review. *PloS one, 12*(12), e0188418.

Brown, R. (2022). 8 Ways to motivate yourself to be healthy. *Psychology Today*. 1 September, 2022. www.psychologytoday.com/gb/blog/understanding-health-behaviors/202209/8-ways-motivate-yourself-be-healthy (last accessed 29th October 2024).

Business of Apps (2025). Wellness App Revenue and Usage Statistics www.businessofapps.com/data/wellness-app-market/ (accessed 28 October 2024)

Casey, K. (2022). *Each day a new beginning: Daily meditations for women*. Mango Media Inc.

Cummins, R. A., Eckersley, R., Pallant, J., Van Vugt, J, and Misajon, R. (2003). Developing a national index of subjective wellbeing: The Australian Unity Wellbeing Index. *Social indicators research, 64*(2), 159–190.

Department of Health. (2011). NHS health and well-being improvement framework. Department of Health.

Devereux, E. (2022). *Allow staff to drink water at nurses' station, England CNO Urges. Nursing Times*. 14 July 2022. Accessed via www.nursingtimes.net/hospital-nursing/allow-staff-to-drink-water-at-nurses-station-england-cno-urges-14-07-2022/ (last accessed 10/2/2025).

Gifkins, J., Johnston, A. and Loudoun, R. (2018). The impact of shift work on eating patterns and self-care strategies utilised by experienced and inexperienced nurses. *Chronobiology international, 35*(6), 811–820.

Gray K. and Tischler, V. (Eds.). (2024). *Creative approaches to wellbeing: The pandemic and beyond*. Manchester University Press.

Huppert, F. A., Marks, N., Clark, A., Siegrist, J., Stutzer, A., Vittersø, J. and Wahrendorf, M. (2009). Measuring well-being across Europe: Description of the ESS well-being module and preliminary findings. *Social Indicators Research, 91*(3), 301–315.

Jackson, S. E., Brown, J., Shahab, L., McNeill, A., Munafò, M. R. and Brose, L. (2023). Trends in psychological distress among adults in England, 2020-2022. *JAMA network open, 6*(7), e2321959–e2321959.

Kagan, I., Ziv, A., Rubin, C., Murad, H., Valinsky, L., Asman, O., Tabak, N. and Wilf Miron, R., (2022). Effect of ethnicity, country of origin and workplace on health behaviors and health perception among nurses: Cross-sectional study. *Journal of Nursing Scholarship, 54*(5), pp. 535–545.

Kleiner, S. M. (1999). Water: An essential but overlooked nutrient. *Journal of the American Dietetic Association*, *99*(2), 200–206.

Koob, G. F. (2024). Alcohol use disorder treatment: Problems and solutions. *Annual Review of Pharmacology and Toxicology*, *64*(1), 255–275.

Lau, A. L., Cummins, R. A. and McPherson, W. (2005). An investigation into the cross-cultural equivalence of the Personal Wellbeing Index. *Social Indicators Research*, *72*(3), 403–430.

Meier, S. and Stutzer, A. (2008). Is volunteering rewarding in itself? *Economica*, *75*(297), 39–59.

Minshall, D., Tracy, D. K., Tarn, M. and Greenberg, N. (2024). Mental health at work: Societal, economic and health imperatives align; it's time to act. *The British Journal of Psychiatry*, *224*(4), 115–116.

Mosley, M. (2024). Just one thing – with Michael Mosley www.bbc.co.uk/programmes/p09by3yy/episodes/guide (last accessed 10/2/2025)

Nichol, B., Wilson, R., Rodrigues, A. and Haighton, C. (2024). Exploring the effects of volunteering on the social, mental, and physical health and well-being of volunteers: an umbrella review. *Voluntas: International Journal of Voluntary and Nonprofit Organizations*, *35*(1), 97–128.

Osteen, J. (2024). *Your best life now: 7 steps to living at your full potential*. FaithWords. www.reformedreflections.org/book-reviews/your-best-life-now.pdf (last accessed 15.11.2024)

Pérula-Jiménez, C., Romero-Rodríguez, E., Fernández-Solana, J., Fernández-García, J. Á., Parras-Rejano, J. M., Pérula-de Torres, L. Á., . . . and Collaborative Group ALCO-AP20 Study. (2024, January). Primary care professionals' empathy and its relationship to approaching patients with risky alcohol consumption. *Healthcare*, *12*(2), 262). MDPI.

Rohr, R. (2023). *Falling Upward, Revised and Updated: A Spirituality for the Two Halves of Life*. John Wiley & Sons.

Schneider, A., Bak, M., Mahoney, C., Hoyle, L., Kelly, M., Atherton, I. M. and Kyle, R. G. (2019). Health-related behaviours of nurses and other healthcare professionals: A cross-sectional study using the Scottish Health Survey. *Journal of Advanced Nursing*, *75*(6), 1239–1251.

Sharma, I., Marwale, A. V., Sidana, R. and Gupta, I. D. (2024). Lifestyle modification for mental health and well-being. *Indian Journal of Psychiatry*, *66*(3), 219–234

Shirreffs, S. M. and Maughan, R. J. (1997). Restoration of fluid balance after exercise-induced dehydration: Effects of alcohol consumption. *Journal of Applied Physiology*, *83*(4), 1152–1158.

Subhani, M., Dhanda, A., Olaru, A., Dunford, L., Ahmad, N., Wragg, A., Frost, K., Greenwood, J., King, M., Jones, K.A. and Rosenberg, W. (2024). Top ten research priorities for alcohol use disorder and alcohol-related liver disease: results of a multistakeholder research priority setting partnership. *The Lancet Gastroenterology & Hepatology*, *9*(5), pp. 400–402.

Tate, C., Wang, R., Akaraci, S., Burns, C., Garcia, L., Clarke, M. and Hunter, R. (2024). The contribution of urban green and blue spaces to the United Nation's sustainable development goals: an evidence gap map. *Cities*, *145*, 104706.

Waldinger, R. (2016). *What makes a good life? Lessons from the longest study on happiness*. Ted Talk: accessed via www.youtube.com/watch?v=8KkKuTCFvzI (last accessed 10/2/2025).

Chapter 11

Workplace well-being

We are not finished yet

Sally Hardy

INTRODUCTION

Understanding workplace well-being has taken us through a process of discovery, personally and professionally, within each chapter of this book. At the start, consideration was given to what health, wealth and happiness means, then chapters have moved through career development as a leader, to personal physical and mental well-being strategies, alongside what structured services and other workplace well-being initiatives can provide.

The different chapters have provided learning resources, case studies, research evidence, all with the intention of sparking interest, triggering renewed vigour, to achieve workplace well-being through self-care and self-compassion, which will in turn lead to improved well-being and sustained compassion for others. This final chapter is more about where you wish to go next on your personal and professional workplace well-being experience. We are not finished yet. You are a work in progress, a lifelong journey of self-discovery, potentials and growth. Having made it to the last chapter of this book, it is now over to you to take the next steps to being who you want to be and knowing how you want to get there.

Bear Grylls (2012), an ex-soldier and survival specialist, says, 'Like you, I am still a work in progress, but I am trying, like you, to do better. Every day a little kinder, a little more generous, and taking myself a little less seriously' (Grylls, 2012: Chp 32).

A WORK IN PROGRESS

Looking after ourselves is a great starting point for well-being (Hardy and Dwaah, 2023). Having been brought up a female, daughter, sister, mother, aunt, etc., I have been socialized into providing and caring for others, with rarely a thought to what

DOI: 10.4324/9781041057956-12

my own body, mind and well-being required. I have learnt this is not sustainable. I need to rest (i.e., sleep), refuel, as in good food and laughter, and I need recuperation time for hobbies, friends and holidays. I also need my friends and family to restore me, as this level of social connection feeds my soul. It is now over to you to take what you have read into your working lives and into your home life. Taking it step by step towards change for the better is about allowing yourself to become important, if not central in sustaining how to care with compassion.

LEARNING RESOURCE

What is it you need, and what is missing in your life that will sustain you?

Try undertaking the life wheel, attributed to Paul J Meyer (1960s), as a technique to help consider where you are now, what aspects of your life you might wish to grow and give more energy and time to.

Draw a circle and divide into a maximum of twelve slices.

Identify the different pieces with key areas of your life, in terms of *personal relationships*, *career*, *physical health*, *finances*, *spirituality*, *parenting*, *home life*, *mental health*, *hobbies*, etc., labelling whatever it is that is important to you, adding these areas up to the same number of segments required on your life wheel. Then score each of these on a scale of 0–10, placing 0 closest to the centre of the circle, 10 at the outer, and then create a spider diagram connecting each. See subsequent example from Stopforth (2022).

EVERY DAY A LITTLE KINDER

There is a world kindness day (13th November) every year, when people are encouraged to undertake a small act of kindness, to pause and consider the value of kindness.

A website dedicated to Random Acts of Kindness, www.randomactsofkindness.org, identifies simple activities to make kindness a normal, everyday intervention with others. However, kindness often starts within and being able to be kind to your 'self'.

Acts of self-kindness involves having to forgive our inherent flaws, failings, mistakes, inadequacies and allow space for self-compassion. This is not about just sailing through life saying 'oops, sorry' and then moving on as if nothing or nobody has been affected by our failings, or mistakes; it is more about acknowledging

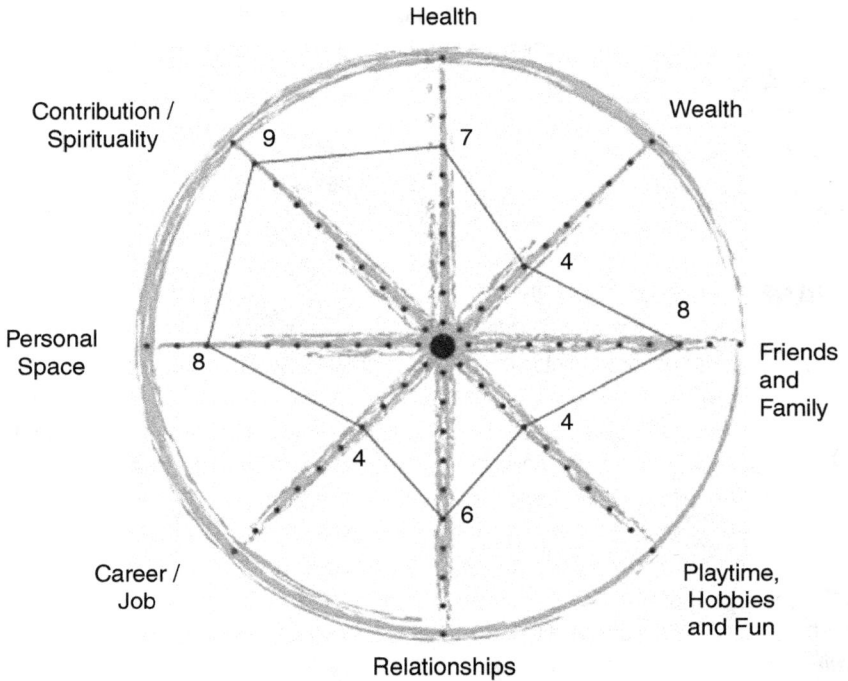

Figure 11.1 Wheel of Life Completed example from Stopforth (2022)

where lessons can be learnt, and where growth and developments need to be taken. Our inner voice, as self-critique, is our harshest enemy, often heard as an internal dialogue we have with ourselves, particularly when trying something new or untested. Within the well-being app industry, there are many free resources that can be used via your phone, laptop or any tablet to address the negative impact self-talk can have on our mental health, and provide resources for addressing a more positive shift in how we talk to and think about ourselves.

Practicing gratitude is another tool that helps refocus our attention away from negativity, and more towards identifying and acknowledging positives. Reframing our thinking is one step towards strengthening our minds, and being prepared for the day or stressful events that can suddenly crash into us or have, over the years, crept up on us.

REFLECTION

- Take time to reflect each day on what you are grateful for.
- Reflect on what and where you did a good job.

- Who was important in supporting you that day?
- Write/capture these reflections in a journal, or start an appreciation jar as thoughts, feelings, activities.
- Look back at what you have written, drawn, or captured.
- Can you see a change, or pattern, in how and whether you are coping?
- Can you identify where and how you can alter your approach?
- Send thank-you notes and cards, or write your partner, or kids, love notes in appreciation of what they bring to your life.
- When people send thank-you cards, store them so that when you are feeling pressurized, or particularly alone, you can be reminded of how much you mean to others.

I used to keep a folder on my laptop at work to store the positive and constructive feedback I received, so that when I was made to think I was not performing, or didn't get the job I was going for, I could remind myself and balance out those negative, imposter syndrome ways of seeing myself.

Ann Frank (1942–1944), whose diaries have become famous, wrote when she was a 13-year-old during war time occupation:

> How lovely to think that no one need wait a moment. We can start now. Start slowly changing the world. How lovely that everyone, great and small can make their contribution toward introducing justice straightaway. . . . And you can always, always give something, even it if is only kindness.

Some interesting research has shown that teams with high levels of agreeableness (openness, conscientiousness) improve team performance, particularly when there is a high level of task uncertainty (Lim et al., 2023). In other words, teams that spend time getting to know each other, are kind and get on well, show mutual respect for each other, often share the same values (kindness as a virtue to be shared in the workplace) are more likely to support and enable each other to overcome workplace stressors.

A little more generous

Generosity is often defined as the habit of giving without anticipation of receiving anything in return. It has long been recognized that human beings are generous creatures. We support each other, provide our time, donate money and share our expertise with others, often for no personal gain other than through a deeply motivated sense of enhanced connection with others. In the first chapter we explored happiness, and the benefits of positive emotions, outcomes and satisfaction this brings as a subjective aspect of well-being. Helping others (as well as ourselves) is voluntary, yet research indicates it is more complex than this.

Three key elements are important to consider when being generous to others, through the self-determination theory (Ryan and Deci, 2024):

1) Autonomy – is this act of generosity a personal choice?
2) Competence – am I able to offer something that is within my ability and areas of interest, or expertise?
3) Relatedness – am I helping this person because I want to have a meaningful relationship with them, or to get closer to this person?

When any one of these three elements are dominant, then the act of generosity can become manipulative. In the modern age, we have to be so careful of grooming behaviours and coercion. It is important to understand the motivation behind any acts of generosity, to ensure the recipient and indeed we ourselves are not being manipulated.

A number of workplaces organize fundraising activities and sports events where money is raised for charity, or specific equipment, arranged as a team building activity. Being asked to donate to charity, or engage in these sorts of events, it is imperative that people have the choice as to what, how and when they wish to donate their time or money to others. Many social problems can be overcome when people come together and work to overcome these in an informed and agreed way such as addressing the rising concerns around loneliness and social isolation in our local neighbourhoods.

Taking myself less seriously

What does it mean to be able to laugh at oneself? The act of laughter is known to improve our immune system, release tense muscles, enhance endorphin release and may even help you live longer. Enjoying yourself, and being able to be self-effacing, allows you to look kindly on yourself and helps maintain a healthy balance between self-centeredness and self-acceptance. Being able to laugh at a situation can build bridges between people. It can bring a levelling element to a highly charged situation. To be able to enjoy life often means not taking everything too seriously.

But laughing at someone is uncomfortable and detrimental. It can be highly offensive to laugh at someone, which may also reveal a level of emotional trauma somewhere in the person's interactions and behaviours. Getting the balance right is important. Think through the intention behind a joke being made. Nervous laughter is often a defense mechanism and an attempt to mask or hide true emotional response. And yet, they say laughter is the best medicine, so laugh often and allow yourself to laugh at your own mishaps and misdemeanors. It's a healthy perspective on life and breeds gratitude, appreciativeness and humility.

A WORKPLACE WELL-BEING CHECKLIST

As the book comes to its conclusion, here is a final checklist to use whenever you need to reconsider what it is you require to check in with yourself and sustain your well-being.

Add in other activities as they emerge that have been useful. You can share these with others on your workplace well-being discovery journey.

Table 11.1 A workplace Well-being checklist

Activity	Well-being	What is required	What to do next
Effective line management processes(	Contribution and role clarity at work alleviates stress response	Regular check-ins, annual appraisal and personal and professional goal setting	If you have not got a regular meeting scheduled, ask for these to be diarized. If you do not have a line manager, seek out someone you can learn from who will provide you with balanced feedback.
Annual leave/ holiday entitlement	Work-life balance	Discuss your holiday plans with family/partner, etc., and book these in the diary/ and get these requests into the roster early.	Schedule regular breaks and plan your annual leave to try to plot these so they fall regularly and are spread out throughout the year

(Continued)

Table 11.1 (Continued)

Activity	Well-being	What is required	What to do next
Know your rights	Support and enablement	Use HR platforms and employee services as required. Ensure you have union representation, and know who/which union is recognized in your organization. Make the most of any professional organizations, such as the UK's Nursing and Midwifery Council or your own Professional Council membership.	Read the policies and procedures. Seek employee assistance advice as required. Keep up to date with mandatory training and any other training on offer to suit your professional and personal development needs.
Budgeting and financial planning	Financial well-being	Manage your money so that stress is reduced, and you are not overstretching your income Undertake an audit of your spending against income. Seek financial or budgeting advice if things are getting out of hand with debt, etc.	Undertake an annual financial planning or budget meeting with your bank. Take out only enough cash for the week, and avoid splashing out on a credit card, to kickstart attempts to save money each month where possible. What pension are you paying into, and what are your retirement plans?

(Continued)

Table 11.1 (Continued)

Activity	Well-being	What is required	What to do next
Team work makes the dream work	Social connections	Spend time getting to know your work colleagues as people. Book to spend time with friends and family to counterbalance time spent at work.	Create a talent board identifying the team's interests, strengths and skills. What work events are taking place that might offer new networking opportunities? Donate some of your time to local community events to get to know people in your hometown/ neighbourhood.
Mental health	Resilience, coping and self-compassion	Stress management Mental health awareness Mindfulness activities	Consider taking up creative journalling or regular journalling of issues as they arise, and learn about how you addressed and managed these over time. Undertake some trainings on offer, such as mental health awareness. Do something physical, like intentional breathing, going for a brisk walk or seeking out a trusted colleague to do a debrief together.

(Continued)

Table 11.1 (Continued)

Activity	Well-being	What is required	What to do next
Physical health	Staying healthy	Menopause awareness Sleep pattern and habits Eat well Drink well	If working remotely and desk bound, make sure you get up and move regularly. Do a workspace ergonomic assessment. Stay hydrated and take care of you.

Source: **Sally Hardy**

CONCLUSION

An average working life is 90,000 hours over a lifetime, or one-third of our life. Then we spend, on average, managing 56 interruptions per day, 304 emails, nearly nine hours per week responding to emails, attend 62 meetings per month and 5.4 hours on unpaid overtime activities (AHRI, 2023). Taking control of your working life and identifying your most productive times, methods and approaches will help provide a balance to the ever-increasing demands of working life.

We then sleep for, on average, 2,229.961 hours in our lifetime, if we get our full eight hours a day. This means we have, on average, 20% of our lives for leisure time. This can get crowded out with children, relatives and other responsibilities like washing, cooking, cleaning. Basically, what this means is use your time wisely. Make time work for you.

A recent podcast I listened to said it takes only eight minutes with a friend or trusted colleague to change our mindset (Sinek, 2024). In other words, you do not need to be spending an agonizing amount of time seeking support for yourself, or feeling guilty for taking five minutes out of a busy schedule to re-focus and address the issues ahead of you.

Prioritize what is important. Set time aside to dedicate to things that bring you joy. Have a diverse set of interests and activities, and choose what best suits your mood, energy levels or comfort needs at that time. Integrate hobbies, interests and enjoyment with your working life. And learn to mentally prepare, mentally rest and mentally engage fully in making the most of what life offers. We are able to set goals, and we are able to learn, grow and give back. So to conclude, achieving workplace well-being is a marathon, not a sprint; therefore we are not finished yet . . .

REFERENCES

Australian HR Institute. (2023) *Infographic. How we spend our time at work*. 18 December 2023. Available via www.hrmonline.com.au/productivity/infographic-how-we-spend-our-time-at-work/ (last accessed 18/2/2025).

Frank, A. (2019) *The Diary of a Young Girl*. The definitive edition. Translated by Susan Massotty, Edited by Otto Frank and Mirjam Pressler. Penguine Modern Classics.

Grylls, B. (2012) *A Survival Guide for Life: How to Achieve Your Goals, Thrive in Adversity, and Grow in Character* (1st Edition). William Morrow. ISBN10: 0062271954

Hardy, S. and Dwaah, M. (2023) looking After Ourselves: Wellbeing, Resilience, and Self-help Strategies. *Chapter 20 in Working With Serious Mental Illness: A Manual for Clinical Practice*, 261.

Lim, S. L., Bentley, P. J., Peterson, R. S., Hu, X. and Prouty McLaren, J. (2023). Kill chaos with kindness: Agreeableness improves team performance under uncertainty. *Collective Intelligence*, 2(1). https://doi.org/10.1177/26339137231158584

Ryan, R. M. and Deci, E. L. (2024) Self-determination theory. In *Encyclopedia of quality of life and well-being research* (pp. 6229–6235). Cham: Springer International Publishing.

Sinek, S. (2024) *It means I need you: The power of 8 minutes*. January 2024 www.youtube.com/watch?v=2lH6x5znOGI (last accessed 18/2/2025)

Stopforth, M. (2021) *The Wheel of Life – a psychologically informed coaching tool?* The Coaching Psychology Network. Updated 7th September 2022. Accessed via www.schoolofcoachingpsy+chology.com/post/the-wheel-of-life-a-psychologically-informed-coaching-tool (last accessed 17/2/2025).

Index

Note: Page numbers in *italics* indicate a figure and page numbers in **bold** indicate a table on the corresponding page.

activity(ies): creative 4, 130, 136–138; generosity 176; kindness 174; physical 76, 132, 145, 158; self-care 16, 38; social 16; stress reducing 13–14; workplace 4, **177–179**

addictive behaviours *see* gambling

Alilyyani, B. 37

Aloweni, F. 52

artificial intelligence (AI) 38, 158

authenticity 76, 79; and integrity 68, 71; in leadership 34, 36–37, 70; self-efficacy 34, 36–37

autonomy 54, 59, 136, 164, 176

awareness 45; creative 134; mindfulness 147; self 53, 56, 76, 130, 152, 166

Axatova, D. 165

Axatova, X. 165

Baker, F. 92

Ball, J. 149, 150

Barnes, A. 114

Basford, J. 130

Bertrand, K. 121

Biriowu, C. 35

Bolton, K. A. 158

Bracht, E. M. 31

British Psychological Society (BPS) COVID-19 guidance 85–86; implementation 86–87; individual well-being 89; SSS approach 88–89; staff support in practice 88

Brown, R. 167

Buchan, J. 149

Bungay, H. 130

burnout 8, 51, 67, 73, 81, 106; likelihood of 39; prevention 49, 52, 55–57, 61, 77, 86; risk of 13, 106

Bush, S. 33

Canzan, F. 105, 106

career 142, 154; adequate staffing levels 151–152; advancement 150; case study 1 143–145; case study 2 146; education opportunities 150; finances 153; healthcare workforce 148–150; self-assessment quiz 147–148; menopause support 152; new staff support 152; reflection task 153–154; supportive leadership and management 151; supportive workplace culture 151; well-being 152–153

Carpenter, B. W. 39

case studies: career 143–146; compassionate leadership 49–51; gambling addiction 112–114; healthy living 159–169; leadership 74–75; mindfulness 146–147; psychological well-being 83–85, 143–145; Schwarts Rounds 100–102; self-care 159–160; self-efficacy 29–30; workplace culture 11–12

Centre for Interprofessional Education (CAIPE) 107

challenge(s): authentic leadership 36–37; compassion and 52–53; of complicated systems 45; leaders' self-care 38–39; Schwartz Rounds 105–106; workforce, healthcare 35–36, 45, 105–107

checklist 5, 89, 151; well-being 91, **91–92**; workplace well-being 177, **177–180**

choice(s) 61, 115, 176; career 75, 105; education 122; healthy 112, 162–163, **168**, **169**; life 123, 163

Coimbra, B. M. 51

compassion(ate) 4, 48–49, 52–55, 61; case study 49–50; challenges 52–53; COVID-19 impact 51–52; culture 106, 109; and empathy 73, 100, 104; leadership 49–51, 59–61, 73–74, 77; reflective task 55; Schwartz Rounds 98; social encounters 106; suicide prevention 48–49, 58–59; *see also* self-compassion

competence 12, 30–32, 60, 176

Coulson, P. 133

counselling 10, 18, 120, 123

COVID-19: aftermath of 51, 85; BPS guidance (*see* British Psychological Society (BPS) COVID-19 guidance); case study 49; consequences of 4, 13, 50; 'frontline' carers 114; health and care staff morale 48, 81; impact on burnout and resilience 51–52; impact on health and well-being 51–52; post era 37, 39, 49, 51; research 51

creativity 128–130, 138–139; activities 137–138; nature, being in, 134–137; photography 134–137; pottery/clay 131–133; websites 139–140

culture: compassionate 106, 109; creative 130; negative social 151; of sharing 105; supportive 151; well-being 123; workplace 2–3, 11–12, 13, 36, 58–59, 78, 150

Cummings, G. 37

Dagogo, E. L-J. 35

Datta, B. 37

Department of Clinical Health Psychology (DCHP) 85

Diagnostic and Statistical Manual of Mental Disorders-5 (DSM-5) 115

diet 161–165; *see also* healthy living

distress 53, 91, 94, 158; moral 51, 57

Dubey, P. 28

Dweck, C. S. 77

Dwyer, L. P. 28

Eckert, J. 39

Egan, H. 53, 57

emotion(s/al) 4, 70, 98: compassion (*see* compassion(ate)); distress (*see* distress); exhaustion 51; happiness (*see* happiness); intelligence 72, 73, 130, 133, 150; positive 175; regulation 76; resilience (*see* resilience); self-care **42–43**, 100; sharing 97; stress (*see* stress); trauma 176–177; well-being 77, 88–89, 100, 137

empathy 55; and compassion 73, 100, 104; fatigue 56; in leadership 73, 76; personal and professional lives 67; self-care 112

empowerment 12, 130, 136

environment: care 142, 166; collaborative 73; safe 98, 99; supportive 60, 73; sustainability 10; technological and intellectual 36; workplace 28, 31, 34–35, 37–38, 75, 147, 153, 165

exercise, physical 14, 76, 145

family 15, 39, 77, 153, 162; feedback 11; learning resources 166–167; leave policies 10; psychological care 88

finances(ial) 8, 11, 121, 164, 173; planning **178**; renumeration 153; stress 10, 114, 115; wellbeing 121, 164

Firth-Cozens, J. 83

Francis, L. 33

Frank, A. 175

Freshwater, D. 133

friends 15, 16, 18, 77, 91, 122, 121, 122

Gabriel, P. I. 35

gambling 112–117, 120–121; case study 112–114; budgeting and financial management 122; contingency management (CM) 122; disorder, DSM-5 115; education 122–123; person-centred gambling severity gauge 120, *120*, 121; self-help strategies 117, 120–121; shame and stigma 121–122; risk with friends 121; toolkits and tips for behaviour change 123; treatment options 117, **118–119**

Gardner William, L. 37
Garside, J. 149, 150
generosity 175–176
Gibbs, G. 102
Gilbert, P. 52, 53
goals 8, 11, 15, 16, 36, 76, 152, 165; setting 166, **169**
Grant, L. 52
Greenberg, N. 51
growth mindset 15, 77

habits: changing 165; development 18; eco-friendly 165; generosity 175; healthy lifetime 5; physical 158; self-care 39
happiness 2, 8–9, 18, 163–165; global public policy and economic impact on 9–11; theoretical foundation 18, **19–24**; *see also* self-care
health 7–8, 18; global public policy and economic impact on 9–11; happiness and 9; *see also* self-care
healthy living 158–159, 165–166; case study 159–169; happiness 163–165; diet 163–165; drinking 162–163; eating 161–162; learning resources 166–167, **168–170**; reflection 160–161; sustainable life 165–166
helping 14, 39, 55, 59, 107, 159, 176; gamblers 117, 121; well-being 137
Hoang, G. 33, 34
Hughes, V. 34
humanity 56, 57, 61, 97, 98

inspire(ing) 38, 59, 70, 71, 72, 136, 142
integrity 34, 61, 67; lacking 71; in leaders 69, 71, 72; leading well 68

Jackson, A. 4
Jafarinia, S. 38
John, S. 31

Kabat-Zinn, J. 76
Kane, A. 40
kindness 5, 98, 173–175; activities 174; care with 73–74; in leadership 77; in values-driven leadership 77; *see also* self-kindness
Kinman, G. 52, 57, 60, 83, 89
Kouzes, J. M. 76
Krampitz, J. 32

Lartey S. A. 28
leadership: adaptive 69; authenticity 34, 36–37, 70; case study 29, 74–75; challenges 31, 33, 34–37, 38; compassionate 49–51, 59–61, 73–74, 77; complexities 69–70; effective 67–68; expectations balance 37–38; factors affecting **33**; feedback 74–75; integrity 71–72; kindness in 77; multidimensionality 32–33; personal growth 76–77; professionalism 72; self-efficacy 28, 30–32; supportive networks 44–45; toolkit 77–79; type of 68–69; *see also* self-efficacy; self-care
learning 2, 10; continuous 17, 45, 69, 77, 154; creative 129, 133–134; interactive approaches 74; interprofessional 103; and opportunities 32; from practice 83; reflective activity 53, 102; resources 2, 5, 56, 122–123, 172, 173; shared 133
Lee, C. 32
loneliness 161, 176
Luu, T. T. 33, 34
Lydgate, J. 79

Marufu, T. 149
meaning: eudaimonic well-being 8; and purpose 105; sense of 91; through creativity 4, 129–133
mental health 59, 76, 115, 136, 174, **179**; of health professions 48–50, 88; issues 51, 53–54, 114, 163; older people's 130; physical exercise 145; public policies 10; stress and 82, 94, 105; support 18, 61; treatments 158
Meyer, P. J. 173
Michalek, D. 33
mindfulness 7, 76, 83, 123; awareness 147; based cognitive therapy 13; of self-compassion 56, 57
Moe, M. 31
Mosley, M. 162
Mowbray, D. 83

National Health Service (NHS) 81; Check study 82; Education for Scotland (2020) 89, 90, **91–92**; employee suicide 58; employers (2024) 106; long-term plan (2019) 117; Long Term Workforce Plan (2023) 48, 149; National Suicide

Prevention Toolkit for England 58;
People Promise (2024) 105; Well-Being
Framework (2021) 48
National Institute for Health and Care
Excellence (NICE) 164
nature, being in, 134–137; *see also* creativity
Noise, H. 130
nutrition *see* healthy living

opportunity(ies): challenges as 15;
educational 32, 77, 129, 133, 143,
150; factors affecting leadership **33**;
financial stability 8; for growth 9, 38, 78;
professional 10, 2, 38, 150
Osteen, J. 166

Pachi, A. 114
Pathak, A. K. 28
peer support 86, 88, 117, 124, 151
physical: activity 14, 76, 132, 145, 158;
environment 164; health 2, 57, 76, 77,
85, 114, 123, 130, 152, 164, 173, **180**; risk
factors 13; self-care **41**; well-being 7–8,
76, **90**, **91–92**, 134, 163, 172; workplace
environment 38
Point of Care Foundation (PoCF) 98, 100, 109
policies: development 49; family leave 10;
public 7, 9–10; well-being 83; in workplace
14, 58
Posner, B. Z. 76
post-traumatic stress disorder (PTSD) 82, 86
Pressley, C. 149, 150
professionalism 69, 72, 74, 76, 79
psychological well-being 81–83, 94–95; case
study 84–85; first-aiders 93–94; group
resilience program 92–93; secondary
intervention 89, **90**, 91, **91–92**; staff
support, hospital based 85; primary
intervention 88–89; tertiary intervention
93; *see also* British Psychological Society
(BPS) COVID-19 guidance

reflection: art-based research 133–136;
effective leadership 68, 79; gambling
severity gauge 121; from practice 74;
retention strategies 147–148, 153–154;
Schwartz Rounds 99–100; self 5, 14,
16, 67, 123; self-care through creativity
136–137; well-being 93, 160–161,
174–175; workplace stressors 14–15

relatedness **168**, 176
resilience 17, 51, 76, 83, 152–153; clinical
pathways 121; COVID-19 impact on
51–52; group program 92–93; skills 89, 91,
164; workforce 4
reward(s) 86, 99, 105–106, 149–150
Richardson, M. 137
Rogers, R. 115
Rohr, R. 166

Sahu, K. K. 28
Sandford, H. 4, 134, 138
Saxena, P. 53
Schuler, A. 117
Schwartz, K. 4, 98–109
Schwartz Rounds 98–100, 108–109; case
study 100–102; challenges and rewards,
healthcare work 105–106; facilitators and
barriers in 107–108; in higher education
103–105; reflection 99–105
self-assessment 11, 14; career 147–148;
happiness 18, **19–22**; self-care 41,
41–44; workplace tools and well-being
approaches **23–24**
self-care 15–16, 38–39; case study 159–160;
creativity 136–137; emotional **42–43**,
100; empathy 112; habits 39; journaling
17; leadership 38–39, *39–40*; physical **41**;
psychological **41–42**; reflective exercise
17–18, 39–40; self-assessment 41, **41–44**;
self-confidence 40; spiritual 43; strategies
16–17; workplace **43–44**
self-compassion 55–57; balanced approach
77; burnout prevention 55–58, 61;
humanity 56, 57; mindfulness of 56, 57; in
practice 52–55; reflective task 57
self-efficacy 28; authenticity 34, 36–37; case
study 29; leadership 28, 30–32; *see also*
leadership
self-kindness 56, 57; in well-being 4,
49, 173, **179**; in workplace 52–55, 172;
see also compassion(ate); *see also*
kindness
Sengupta, P. 53
sharing *see* Schwartz Rounds
Siciliano, M. D. 44
Sinclair, S. 53
sleep 91, 145, 173, 180; patterns 5, 158;
problems 86; in shift workers 89;
workplace retention 152

social: activities 16; care 1, 4, 12, 13, 45, 60, 73, 81–82, 97, 100, 103–106, 142, 150, 152, 154; challenges 58; culture 151; encounters 97–109; environment 9; well-being 7, **90**, **91–92**

staff: burnout 106; care 38, 48, 81; checklist 151; emotions of 53; health 48, 58, 82, 164; migration 34–35; motivation 37; NHS 34–35, 59, 81–82, 94; support hospital-based service 83, 85, 87; well-being 51, 83–85, 100, 143–145; workplace culture 4, 11–12

staff support service (SSS) 4, 92, 93, 95; during Covid-19 pandemic 83–85, 87; hospital-based service 85; visible leadership, importance of 88–89

Steptoe, A. 9

Stickley, T. 133

stigma 10, 115, 121

Stopforth, M. 173

strategies: compassion and self-compassion 48, 61; retention 147, 150; self-care 15, 16, 18; self-help 117, 120–121; staff in health and social care 150; workplace well-being 5, 57

stress 1, 14–15, 39, 56, 58–59, 100, 114; financial 10; management 18, 76, 150; and mental health 82; physical 15; and poorer well-being 88; reduction 76–77

suicide prevention 4, 49–50, 58–59, 61, 120

support(ing): culture 151; environment 60, 73; friends 15, 91; gambling treatment 117; leadership 44–45, 59, 151;

networks 14–15; peer 117; policies 10; psychological 18, 59, 61, 85, 93; staff 4, 48, 82–85, 87; well-being at work 1–2, 51, 91, **91–92**, 104, 106, 109

sustainability 4, 10, 104, 149, 165–166

Teoh, K. 83, 89

Thomas, B. 117

Urick, A. 39

Vella Burrows, T. 130

wealth 7–8; global public policy and economic impact 9–10

websites, creativity 139–140

well-being, workplace 1–2, 172–173, 180–181; case study 11–12; checklist 177, **177–180**; culture 11–12; generosity 175–176; kindness 173–174; laughter 176–177; learning resources 173–174, *174*; reflection 174–175; shared purpose 12–13; stressors 13–14

wellness programmes 18, 158–159, 166

West, M. 54, 55, 59, 60

West, T. H. 75

Wong Carol, A. 37

workplace wellbeing *see* well-being, workplace

Yang, M. 33, 34

Zarobe, L. 130

Zulueta, P. de 52, 60

For Product Safety Concerns and Information please contact our EU
representative GPSR@taylorandfrancis.com
Taylor & Francis Verlag GmbH, Kaufingerstraße 24, 80331 München, Germany